Managing the
National Health Service

Managing the National Health Service

Shifting the frontier?

Stephen Harrison

Lecturer in Health Services Organisation
Nuffield Institute for Health Services Studies
University of Leeds

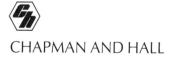

CHAPMAN AND HALL

London · New York · Tokyo · Melbourne · Madras

UK   Chapman and Hall, 2–6 Boundary Row, London SE1 8HN

USA   Chapman and Hall, 29 West 35th Street, New York NY10001

JAPAN   Chapman and Hall Japan, Thomson Publishing Japan, Hirakawacho Nemoto Building, 7F, 1–7–11 Hirakawa-cho, Chiyoda-ku, Tokyo 102

AUSTRALIA   Chapman and Hall Australia, Thomas Nelson Australia, 102 Dodds Street, South Melbourne, Victoria 3205

INDIA   Chapman and Hall India, R. Seshadri, 32 Second Main Road, CIT East, Madras 600 035

First edition 1988
Reprinted 1991

© 1988 Stephen Harrison

Printed in Great Britain by St Edmundsbury Press Ltd
Bury St Edmunds, Suffolk

ISBN 0 412 33960 9

British Library Cataloguing in Publication Data

Harrison, Stephen, 1947–
     Managing the National Health Service:
     shifting the frontier?
     1. Great Britain. National health services. Management
     I. Title
     362.1'068
ISBN 0-412-33960-9

CONTENTS

CONTENTS

TABLES AND FIGURES

Tables

Figures

ACKNOWLEDGEMENTS

It is not possible to spend a decade teaching in a University without either becoming extremely arrogant or acquiring numerous debts to colleagues and students. I cannot mention all these here, but I especially wish to acknowledge the help of Keith Barnard and Jack Hallas (University of Leeds), Chris Ham and David Hunter (King's Fund Institute), Christopher Pollitt (Open University), and Stuart Haywood (University of Birmingham). The Bibliography is testament to my utilisation of the insights of Rudolf Klein, who also read the entire manuscript and made a number of helpful comments. Specific thanks are due to Andrew Green (University of Leeds), Michele Corrado (MORI), Jack Hyde (CBI), Ralph Howell M.P., and Paul Gardner (Conservative Research Department). As noted in Chapter 1 below, the book occasionally draws on data from as yet unreported research projects, and I wish to record my gratitude to all my informants. It is usual for authors to accept responsibility for any errors which have survived the scrutiny of all those who have helped. I do this willingly.

The preparation of the book has been made easier by a number of other people. Without the help of Lorraine Bate, Deborah Raven, Bernadette Shaw, Jean Frame and Elizabeth Breckin, all of the Nuffield Institute Library, I should have spent many more hours of chasing references than I did. Jane Welsh has performed miracles of high-speed wordprocessing in producing the text. And I owe a special debt to my partner, Sally Brown, for her support throughout; it cannot be very stimulating to receive, in answer to a question about what one did today, the reply 'I wrote five pages of Chapter 4.'

Steve Harrison
University of Leeds
Nuffield Institute for Health Services Studies

Chapter 1

THE FRONTIER OF CONTROL

For more than three decades now, the National Health Service (NHS) has been obsessed with notions of 'better management'. Indeed, most commentators are in favour of better management in much the same way as they might oppose sin: as a truism. The sceptical observer, faced with this knowledge and yet seeing the NHS in the throes of yet more managerial reforms, is entitled to ask what, if anything, is different about the Griffiths innovations and other contemporary changes? Chapters 2, 3, and 4, of this book attempt to answer that question by comparing changing conceptions of the desirable role of the NHS manager before and after 1982; the conclusion which is reached is that these recent changes represent the first serious attempt, in the lifetime of the NHS, to shift the 'frontier of control' between, on the one hand, doctors (physicians), and, on the other, the government.

Where do health service managers fit into this? After all it is the relationships between managers and professionals which provide the acid test of any strategy of increasing management control; the mere definitions of 'management' and 'professionalism' are sufficient to sensitise the observer to the potential for conflict. From the aphorism that management is 'getting things done through people' to Fayol's (1971, originally published 1916) classical statement that management consists of planning, organisation, commanding, co-ordination and control, definitions emphasise control over others. This theme is retained in the work of modern management writers such as Drucker (1979 p. 20) and Stewart:

> The manager's job can be broadly defined as deciding what should be done and then getting other people to do it (Stewart 1979 p. 69).

By contrast, definitions of professionalism tend to emphasise autonomy, whether simply as a trait exhibited by certain occupations, whether as something which is functionally desirable in order to allow optimum use of complex knowledge, or whether (more critically) as a strategy by which occupational groups seek to enhance both the economic and qualitative conditions of their employment. (For a discussion, see Johnson 1972).

The medical application of this notion of autonomy is 'clinical freedom' (clinical autonomy). Though doctors are apparently rarely able to articulate a coherent definition of what this constitutes (Harrison et al 1984a), various academic definitions are available. One such definition is that of Tolliday (1978, pp. 41-45), who identifies four kinds of claim to autonomy made by doctors, each cast in terms of freedom from control by particular actors: the right to practise free from hierarchical management; the right to refuse an individual patient; the right to lead and co-ordinate other health professions; and the right to regard medical knowledge as overarching that of other disciplines. An alternative classification, based on doctors' own fragmented notions of what is involved, is that of Schulz and Harrison (1986, pp. 338-340): choice of specialty and practice location; control over earnings; control over the nature and volume of tasks; acceptance of patients; control over diagnosis and treatment; control over the evaluation of care; and control over other professionals. It is evident that the relationships of doctors and managers are potentially crucial determinants of the latter set of components.

But the logic of these definitions does not imply that managers and professionals will always be in conflict. Rather, conflict will only occur when and if the two groups are pursuing differing objectives. Professionals may be perceived as technical experts and managers may be content to assume that professional decisions are the best available; a number of modern theorists of bureaucracy have identified a type of organisation in which, despite being surrounded by overall bureaucratic controls, professionals are substantially left to get on with it (Pugh and Hickson 1976; Mintzberg 1979). Health services can be, and indeed have been, seen as fitting this model; doctors are the archetypal profession.

Twentieth century health services, however, display a characteristic which, it is argued, was bound eventually to render such an arrangement unstable. This can be clarified by comparing the modern medical relationship with the Nineteeenth Century (somewhat idealised) situation upon which notions of medical ethics, and relevant law, are still modelled. (For a critique, see Williams n.d.). The latter relationship involves only the doctor and the patient; the doctor provides advice and/or treatment in return for 'informed consent' to the treatment, and a fee. The only limits on treatment are the doctor's competence on the one part and the patient's consent and resources on the other. Within these limits, the doctor's ethical duty is do his or her absolute best for the individual patient. No question of clinical freedom arises, except insofar as both the parties are entitled to choose to transact, or not. This is characterised in Figure 1.1.

More recent developments in health services have, however, introduced third parties into the relationship. Initially these took the form of owners of hospitals, but with the development of state health services have come third party payers for health care; government itself in countries such as Britain, sick funds in many of the countries of continental Europe, and insurance companies together with a range of government agencies in the United States. To the extent that they meet insurance or fund contributions for their workers, employers too may be regarded as amongst these third parties.

Third party payment for health care, even though it largely consists of the pooling of contributions by taxpayers or the insured population, means that no individual patient has any incentive to restrict the amount of care he or she seeks (moral hazard). Nor is there any such incentive for the provider of care. In the context of what is now the conventional wisdom that demand for health care is unlimited (for the original statement of this position, see Roberts 1952), and the truism that resources are finite, a process of rationing of health care is bound eventually to occur. It is upon the third parties that the incentive to ration falls. In principle, third parties have the option of either or both of rationing the consumer/patient's entitlement (which is what health care insurance policies and charges to patients do),

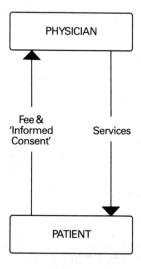

Figure 1.1 The Idealised Liberal Concept of Medicine.

or of controlling the resources for care provided to doctors, and perhaps other professionals for whom doctors act as 'gatekeeper'. The latter option is the only one, in principle, available in a health care system which (like the NHS) purports to be comprehensive, though the anomaly of prescription and dental charges is now of such antiquity that it is scarcely seen as such. Claims to clinical freedom on the part of doctors can be seen as resistance against control over health care providers. This state of affairs is characterised in Figure 1.2.

It is, of course, clear that clinical freedom cannot be absolute (since it would necessarily entail the freedom of one doctor to impinge on the freedom of another), nor is it claimed to be by doctors or anyone else. Rather, it is a question of what restrictions by third parties are considered to be legitimate or illegitimate. It is such perceptions which demarcate the 'frontier of control', a phrase borrowed from the title of Goodrich's classic study of worker-management relationships in Britain in the period immediately following the Great War of 1914-1918. Just as those years were ones of unpreced-ented trade union resistance to management control, so the 1980s have seen unprecedented government resistance to medical domination of the NHS. This book argues that the chosen strategy for this resistance has been to convert NHS managers from agents of medicine to agents of government: to shift their location in terms of Figure 1.2.

Two further questions follow closely from this conclusion, and this book is also concerned with addressing these. Firstly, why have such attempts at controlling doctors arisen just now? The answer offered by Chapters 5 and 6 is complex, involving a range of factors from macroeconomic pressures to changes in the functioning of committees of the House of Commons to current political ideologies. Secondly, an assessment of the impact of the Griffiths and related changes is called for; what are the prospects for a shift in the frontier of control? There are important caveats to be made in connection with this question; the reforms are recent and it may be too early to reach firm conclu-sions, though it should be noted that the short-term contracts given to NHS General Managers (see below, Chapter 4) imply early and visible results. Consequently, the conclusions are tentative and

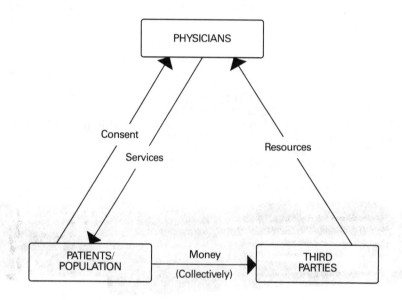

Figure 1.2 The Health Service Model of Medicine

must await confirmation, or otherwise, by the major empirical studies currently being conducted. In the meantime, the answer suggested in Chapter 8 is that the frontier of control between doctors and managers has not yet moved very much, for reasons which are explored, along with some current political developments which might lead to rather greater change in the future.

Neither of these two further questions can be addressed without the employment of theory; both explanation and prediction require some assumptions about how the world 'works'. The view adopted here is that it is better for these assumptions to be made explicit (and therefore challengeable) rather than left implicit: in J.M. Keynes' famous dictum 'Practical men, who believe themselves to be quite exempt from any intellectual influences, are usually the slaves of some defunct economist' (Keynes 1936). A number of references to theories are therefore made in Chapters 3 and 4, culminating in a more extended discussion in Chapter 6. The position reached is that no single theory is adequate for these purposes; to argue, for instance, that the Griffiths developments are simply the product of economic pressure leaves open the explanation of why the developments took the form which they did. Consequently, Chapter 6 discusses a number of theories of different levels of generality, and attempts to link these together.

Most of the themes of this book have been aired, though not fully developed, in earlier publications; such sources are referenced where appropriate. Some readers will find the general level of references irritatingly high and wonder if they are being used as a drunk uses a lamp post: for support rather than illumination. This is partly true, since some of the conclusions are likely to be contentious, but in any event the reader is entitled to embark upon his or her own literature search with the maximum of assistance. One exception to this policy of full referencing occurs because Chapters 5 and 6 make occasional use of unattributable interview material obtained for the purpose of research projects which as yet are unreported.

The overall purpose of this book is to help those who work in the NHS, and those who study it, to understand what is happening and what is likely to happen. For students of social policy, the book provides a case study in one public policy sector of something which is becoming increasingly prominent in other sectors: growing managerialism. The Jarratt Report into the organisation of universities, performance-related pay for schoolteachers, the creation of an Inspectorate for the personal social services, the computerisation of social security calcuations, and the development of 'performance indicators' in the police and prison services can all be seen as part of the same phenomenon, as can the central government Financial Management Initiative. (For a commentary on some of these see Pollitt 1986; Fry 1984).

It should also be made clear what this book is not. It does not examine the process by which the Griffiths Inquiry reached its conclusions, nor does it purport to be a systematic evaluation of the impact of the Griffiths reforms; there are many criteria, other than their impact on doctors, by which these reforms can be judged. The book does not purport to give a detailed account of the creation of the NHS (for which, see Eckstein 1958; Lindsey 1962; Willcocks 1967; Pater 1981), its history (for which see Watkin 1978; Klein 1983), or its detailed structure (for which see the unfortunately slightly dated Levitt and Wall 1984). For analysis of British health policy as a whole, the reader is referred to Ham (1985) or Allsop (1984).

Finally, this book does not constitute either a prescription or a partisan analysis, although 'value-free' social science is certainly a chimera. It is simply not at all self-evident whether or not reductions in clinical freedom, if they occur, will produce more, or less, effective and appropriate health care.

Chapter 2

THE FORMALITIES OF MANAGEMENT AND ORGANISATION

The years from not long after the inception of the NHS in 1948 until 1981 were increasingly occupied by a series of debates about the organisation and management of the Service; some of these resulted in organisational change, others did not. This Chapter summarises these debates and developments; it is a daunting history consisting as it does of innumerable official reports, complex organisation structures, and interminable debate amongst the affected interest groups. The brief account which follows contains only the major features of this history, and is employed to support three propositions:

. successive governments have had no serious aspirations for the control of the medical profession by NHS managers; clinical freedom has been a continuing component of British health policy;
. it has been taken for granted that 'better management' of the NHS would result from improving the lot of NHS managers by such means as improving promotion opportunities; this has provided the opportunity for the professions other than medicine to pursue their own management career arrangements; and
. developments related to the health service consumer have been marginal in relation to developments in management and organisation.

Following a more or less chronological presentation of developments from 1948 to 1982, each of these propositions is discussed in detail.

CHANGING FORMS OF ORGANISATION

The organisational form of the newly-created NHS in 1948 was the 'tripartite' structure, representing a

political compromise between the Labour Government
and the various provider groups. This is summarised
in Figure 2.1. Although services were to be
available to the whole population, General Medical
Practitioners (GPs) remained self-employed contractors to the NHS, remunerated largely through
capitation fees. The contracts of GPs, along with
those of General Dental Practitioners, Pharmacists
and Opticians (also self-employed) were administered
by Executive Councils, upon which the four professions were themselves heavily represented (Lindsey
1962 pp. 82-82). These arrangements were little
more than a continuation of those made in Lloyd
George's National Insurance Act of 1911 (Willcocks
1967 p. 75).

The second arm of the tripartite arrangement was
provided by local government: County Councils and
County Borough Councils. These bodies lost their
duties and rights to provide hospital services,
remaining responsible for preventive services,
maternal and child welfare, health visiting, home
nursing, ambulances, and the School Medical Service
(Levitt 1979 p. 19). Such local authorities
appointed a Health Committee of Councillors, to whom
the Medical Officer of Health (MOH) was responsible
for the above services.

Hospital authorities constituted the third part of
the structure. Great Britain was divided into
nineteen (later twenty) Regions, each containing a
medical school and each controlled by a Regional
Hospital Board (RHB) responsible to the Minister of
Health. Groups of hospitals (occasionally single
large hospitals) within each Region were presided
over by Hospital Management Committees (HMCs) or
Boards of Governors in Scotland. Groups of English
hospitals with medical undergraduate teaching
functions were run by Boards of Governors, who,
unlike HMCs, were responsible not to the RHB but
directly to the Minister of Health. The membership
of Boards and Committees was part-time, honorary,
and appointed rather than elected (see Watkin 1978
pp. 24-26): doctors were heavily represented (Allsop
1984 p. 17). Boards and Committees employed a chief
administrative officer (often known as the Group
Secretary), and individual hospitals were normally
managed on a day to day basis by a triumvirate
consisting of Hospital Secretary, Matron, and
Medical Superintendent or other medically qualified
administrator (Central Health Services Council 1954

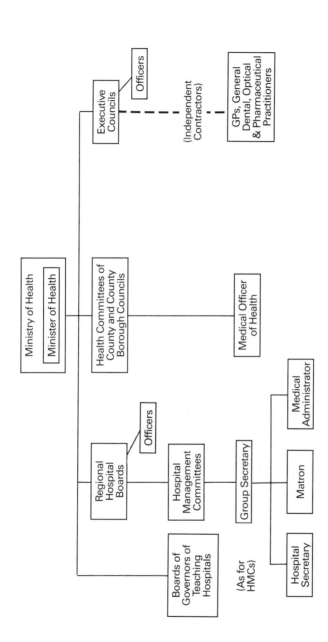

Figure 2.1 Outline Organisational Structure of English NHS; 1948

pp. 12-14). Except in the case of Boards of Governors, Consultants were employed by RHBs rather than HMCs; all Consultants retained their right to engage in private practice by opting for a part-time NHS appointment.

Even before the advent of a Conservative Government in 1951, concern had been growing about the costs of the NHS, which had consistently exceeded estimates (Klein 1983 pp. 33-40). The Guillebaud Committee, established in 1953 to investigate the cost of the NHS, made it clear in its report that there was no financial crisis; rather, estimates had failed to allow for demographic change or the occurrence of inflation. Nevertheless, it went on to call, in very general terms, for more emphasis on 'oversight and supervision of the service' (Committee of Enquiry 1956 para. 211). At roughly the same time, the Bradbeer Committee was responding to the uncertainties about management relationships expressed by NHS managers from widely differing pre-NHS backgrounds. The Committee legitimised the existing trend for HMCs to have one chief administrator at Group level but a triumvirate arrangement at hospital level (see above); it opposed the appointment of matrons or medical officers at group level, and (like Patients First twenty-five years later: see below) argued that lay departmental heads within a hospital should be responsible to the Hospital Secretary (Central Health Services Council 1954, paras. 20, 28, 196). The Noel Hall Report (1957) and the Lycett Green Report (1963) subsequently provided arrangements for the grading, recruitment, training and promotion of NHS Administrative staff (Watkin 1975 pp. 159, 175).

The first decade of operation of the NHS had provided the occasion for the medical profession to call for a review of it; the Porritt Committee produced a wide-ranging Report on behalf of the British Medical Association (BMA) and the Royal Colleges. Notable amongst its recommendations was its call for the integration of the three parts of the tripartite structure, though without changing the employment status of doctors. In each locality the three parts of the service would be separately managed by a medically qualified administrator, though at the level of the individual hospital the Bradbeer recommendations (see above) were endorsed (Medical Services Review Committee 1962, paras. 77,

85, 425). Simultaneous with Porritt's delibera-
tions, the 'Hospital Plan for England and Wales' was
being produced (Ministry of Health 1962); this was
to result in the concept of the 'district general
hospital', offering a comprehensive service from 600
to 800 beds, together with appropriate outpatient
and diagnostic services (Allen 1979 p. 72). It also
provided the occasion for an enhanced management
role in planning and commissioning capital
developments.

The period of Labour Government from 1964 to 1970
was, however, to provide a sustained, if diverse,
emphasis on questions of management. A 1966 paper
on the management functions of hospital doctors
noted that 'the industrial manager works in a....
unified and clear environment; his responsibilities
are.... readily definable and his work is.... easily
evaluated.... . In British hospital management,
these supportive and critical elements are lacking'
(Advisory Committee 1966 pp. 8-9). The paper went
on to urge Consultants to improve management by
improving the scientific scrutiny of their own work
(p. 9). In Scotland, however, the Farquharson-Lang
Report was recommending that RHBs and local
Boards should employ a 'chief executive' and
moreover felt 'reluctantly obliged to disagree with
the conclusion [of the BMA] that the chief executive
... must, inevitably, be a medically qualified
person' (Scottish Health Services Council 1966,
pp. 62-63). Although the Report was publicised in
England, this particular conclusion was not (Watkin
1975 p. 195).

Although Farquharson-Lang had implied that the
desirability of a chief executive was widely
recognised in England, this was not unanimous. In
the same year as Farquharson-Lang, the Salmon
Committee (covering Scotland as well as England)
reported on the subject of a management structure
for senior nursing staff. It concluded that,
notwithstanding Bradbeer (see above), senior nurses
had insufficient status, and went on to propose a
hierarchical structure for the profession, to
include a chief nursing officer at Group level
(Ministry of Health 1966 pp. 4, 60-61). The Salmon
Report was accepted in principle by the Minster and
introduced, initially on a pilot basis, between 1967
and 1972 (Watkin 1975 p. 318). The Mayston Report
soon afterwards applied similar principles to local
authority nurses (Watkin 1978 p. 113).

13

Nevertheless, Farquharson-Lang found some support from south of the border. In what may well have been a reaction against Salmon, a joint working party of the Institute of Hospital Administrators and the King's Fund criticised Bradbeer on different grounds, accusing it of having 'failed to grasp the nettle that someone had to be in command of the [hospital] with authority over all the rest of the staff' (Joint Working Party 1967a p. 24). The report went on to choose the term 'general manager' (pp. 32-34) for such a person, responsible to whom would be, amongst others, a medically qualified Director of Medical and Paramedical Services (p. 38 ff). In what transpired to be a prophetic statement, the Working Party noted that its recommendations might not be immediately acceptable to doctors, and might take fifteen years to come about (p. 42).

During the same period, the medical profession itself had begun to look at the relationship between NHS management and hospital medicine; a joint committee of the Ministry of Health and the profession produced in 1967 the first of three 'Cogwheel Reports' (so named after the logo on their cover), which urged doctors to recognise their essential interdependence with each other and to set up specialty based 'divisions' within hospitals, each sending a representative to a 'Medical Executive Committee'. The Chairman of this latter body would act as the chief medical spokesman (sic) for the hospital or group of hospitals (Joint Working Party 1967b pp. 2-4). The Ministry quickly commended the Report to HMCs and Boards of Governors and medical staff in many districts began to organise themselves either along the lines recommended or some variation of them, though progress was uneven across the country (Watkin 1975 p. 244). Parallel developments occurred in Scotland as a result of the Brotherston Report (Watkin 1975 p. 245-7).

Other health service professions were also interested in management, albeit in a more direct way than the doctors; following Salmon (see above), the Zuckerman (1968) and Noel Hall (1970) Reports recommended management career structures for scientists and technicians, and pharmacists respectively, employed in the NHS (Watkin 1975 pp. 341-349).

The late 1960s also saw the first applications to

the NHS of quantitative management techniques, such as organisation and methods study. Originally used as an aid to planning, such techniques became widespread after 1967 as a means of introducing payment-by-results schemes for hospital manual workers, since current government pay policy required productivity increases in return for pay increases (National Board for Prices and Incomes 1967). Barnard and Harrison (1986 p. 1219) have argued that these developments were a significant spur to increasing levels of trade union membership.

Developments related to the consumer also took place. Following the Howe Report (1967) into the maltreatment of mentally ill and handicapped patients at Ely Hospital in Cardiff, the Hospital Advisory Service (later Health Advisory Service) was established to make periodic assessments of long-stay institutions (Watkin 1978 pp. 78-80). By 1973 a decision had been made to extend the role of the Parliamentary Commissioner ('Ombudsman') to include the NHS, a recommendation originally made in Sans Everything (Abel-Smith 1967), a book which had documented similar allegations in a number of other hospitals (Watkin 1978 pp. 75-78). But these events were all overshadowed by a series of developments which was to culminate in the reorganisation of the NHS in 1974.

It will be recalled that the Porritt Report (see above) had suggested a degree of administrative unification of the tripartite structure of the NHS; also, by the mid-1960s consideration was being given to the reorganisation of local government (Alexander 1982 p. 6). It was not surprising therefore that in 1968 the then Labour Minister of Health, Mr Kenneth Robinson, published a Green Paper (consultative document) on the administrative structure of medical services (Watkin 1975 p. 166). As Klein (1983 p. 90) notes, there was a widespread consensus that greater integration of services was required, together with widespread recognition that medical opposition made the transfer of health services to local government a political impossibility. By later in the same year the Ministry had been amalgamated (also in pursuit of greater integration of social policy) into the new Department of Health and Social Security (DHSS) under Mr Richard Crossman, and in 1970 the latter published a second Green Paper in which it was announced that a reorganisation would take place, with health services (defined in terms of the roles of the health professions) to be administered by (in England) some ninety Area Health Authorities, each sharing boundaries with the local government authority responsible for social services (DHSS 1970 pp. v-vi).

After the election of a Conservative Government in 1970, the new Secretary of State for Social Services, Sir Keith Joseph, published a White Paper (DHSS 1972a) setting out the government's reorganisation intentions; although there were some differences, including the retention of a regional tier of organisation and some explicit references to effective management, the 'successive proposals.... show a remarkable degree of continuity' (Klein 1983 p. 91). Consideration of possible management arrangements had already begun, and by this time there was little, if any, support for the notion of a chief executive officer; intellectual leadership in this area lay in the Health Services Organisation Research Unit at Brunel University, whose members and those influenced by them concluded that doctors could not be made managerially responsible to non-doctors (see, for instance, Jaques 1978 p. 141; Naylor 1971 p. 33). Moreover, by this time the claims of the health professions to managerial roles of their own had been added to by the Hunter Report, which recommended the creation of a new medical specialty of Community Medicine whose responsibilities would include planning and management (Working Party 1972 p. 23). As Lewis (1986 p. 116) puts it, 'doctors had to be persuaded to become actively involved in the management of the service, and it was in this context that the role of the community physician as a "linkman" [sic], inspiring the confidence of both clinicians and administrators, was perceived as crucial.'

It was, however, the so-called 'Grey Book' (DHSS 1972b) which set out the definitive philosophy (even though some of its details in respect of paramedical occupations were later modified) for the management arrangements in the reorganised NHS. Produced by a joint group of DHSS and NHS officers and heavily influenced by the Brunel philosophy (see above) of role clarity within organisations, the Grey Book recommended a system of consensus decisionmaking by multi-disciplinary management teams consisting of administrator, treasurer, nurse, and doctors. The reorganised structure of the NHS was implemented, along with the reorganisation of local government authorities, in April 1974 (by which time a Labour Government had been returned to office), and is summarised in Figure 2.2; for a detailed account see Levitt (1979).

A number of features of the new structure merit comment. Firstly, the principle of non-elected health authorities was preserved, with England divided into fourteen Regions and subdivided into ninety Areas; one departure, however, was the provision for a number of persons appointed by coterminous local authorities to take Area Health Authority membership, and another was the provision of part-time salaries for Authority Chairmen and women. Secondly, rather more than half the Areas were divided into two or more Districts, each nominally based on a district general hospital and with a catchment population sufficient to provide a reasonable range of services. Regional Health Authorities (RHAs) and Area Health Authorities were statutory corporate bodies, whereas the District level was an administrative creation. Thirdly, the contracts of GPs and other independent contractors were held by Family Practitioner Committees (FPCs), established by each Area Health Authority, and consisting of representatives of the relevant professions and of health and local authorities (Levitt 1979 p. 66). Fourthly, a Community Health Council (CHC) was established for each District, outside the line of authority but with the task of representing the views of local health service users. CHC membership was drawn largely from voluntary organisations and local authorities (Levitt 1979 pp. 191 ff).

Management at Regional, Area and District levels was to be conducted by multidisciplinary management teams whose composition is shown in Figure 2.2. Although individual team members were to have personal responsibility for their own spheres of work, issues or decisions which were multidisciplinary or strategic were to be handled collectively. The mode of decisionmaking by such teams was to be consensus, 'that is, decisions ... need the agreement of each of the team members' (DHSS 1972b p. 15; for a review, see Harrison 1982). It should be noted that there was no authority relationship between teams at different levels, only between the Authorities themselves, with team

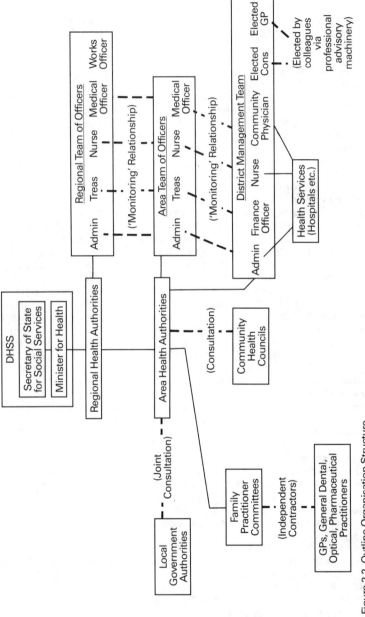

Figure 2.2 Outline Organisation Structure of English NHS; 1974

members responsible to their respective Authorities. Rather, the relationship betweem teams was intended to be one of 'monitoring': the higher level possessing the right to give advice and obtain information but not directly to instruct the lower level (Levitt 1979 p. 48). Disagreements either between teams, or amongst members of a particular team, were to be settled by reference to the appropriate Health Authority, though, as is shown in Chapter 3 below, there was in practice a reluctance to adopt this procedure. In Scotland and Wales, no RHAs were created, and there were some differences of terminology. District teams in these countries were managerially accountable to area teams, and Scottish teams did not include elected clinicians (Levitt 1979 pp. 221-234).

The 1974 reorganisation can also be seen as the culmination of a longstanding trend towards managerial specialisation. Specialist finance and supplies officers had emerged during the 1950s and 1960s, as had specialist managers in such areas as catering, laundry, and domestic work in a period when nurses were increasingly seeking to shed responsibility for 'non-nursing duties'. The professional building and engineering ('Works') function had also developed along with the increasing complexity of health building and technology. In the late 1960s and early 1970s specialist planners and personnel officers had been employed in response, respectively, to activity generated by the Hospital Plan (see above) and to increasing trends in unionisation and employment legislation (Barnard and Harrison 1986 p. 1220). Reorganisation formalised this trend and added to it managerial hierarchies in a number of health professions not already thus organised: dentistry, chiropody, speech therapy, physiotherapy, occupational therapy and dietetics (Levitt 1979 p. 144 ff).

The 1974 Reorganisation was completed by the introduction in 1976 of a planning system. This took a cyclical format. DHSS guidelines on national policies and resource assumptions were issued to RHAs, amplified by them and issued to Area Health Authorities, again amplified and issued to District Management Teams (DMTs) who were then responsible for preparing a district operational plan; the resulting plan was fed upwards for approval or review at Area level, aggregated into Area plans fed to Region, and into Regional plans fed to DHSS (DHSS 1976). The system, though it involved a good deal of consultation with various interests as well as the opportunity for plans at a higher level to be amended as a result of comments from the lower, can be seen as a variety of classic chain-of-command management.

Although substantial numbers of NHS professionals and managers had benefitted considerably from the introduction of the new structure, there was a degree of disillusionment at its complexity and at what proved to be difficult relationships between the various levels of organisation (Ham 1985 p. 30). Moreover the period after 1974 was a difficult one for the NHS for other reasons. Firstly, it was a period of relative economic restraint; in 1976 the Treasury introduced the 'cash limits' system of financial allocation to the public sector. This replaced the previous system of allocation in volume terms and meant that NHS hospital and community health services (though not Family Practitioner Services) were no longer automatically protected against inflation in the costs of its manpower or other resources (Klein 1983 p. 109). A system of central control of management costs was also introduced (Levitt and Wall 1984 p. 60). The introduction in 1978 of the formula for resource allocation devised by the Resource Allocation Working Party ('RAWP') was intended to procure an equitable geographical distribution of health care resources; its application in a period of financial restraint necessarily entailed a redistribution from some health authorities to others. (For a detailed account see Jones and Prowle 1984 pp. 93-99). Secondly, it was a period of increased militancy amongst trade unionists in the NHS; industrial action became relatively commonplace (Barnard and Harrison 1986 p. 1220). Thirdly, between 1974 and 1976 the Government and medical profession were involved in what Klein (1983 p. 117) describes as 'the most bitter political struggle since the inception of the NHS': the battle over an attempt to remove private beds from NHS hospitals. (For a detailed account, see Klein 1980). Against this background the Royal Commission on the National Health Service was established in 1976 under the Chairmanship of Sir Alec Merrison.

By the publication of the Commission's Report in July 1979, a new Conservative government had been elected; the Conservative Party has remained in office since. Like Guillebaud (see above), the Royal Commission was broadly satisfied with the performance of the NHS, though it made a large number of somewhat piecemeal recommendations. Major proposals included the abolition of either the Area or District tier (unspecified) of organisation (Royal Commission 1979 p. 331), the abolition of FPCs (p. 331), and a strengthening of CHCs (p. 157). It also recommended the introduction of a limited list of drugs available for prescription on the NHS (p. 89) though this was soon rejected by the Secretary of State (DHSS 1979a).

A good deal of the Government response to the Report was contained in Patients First, a consultative document published in December 1979; this document proposed the abolition of the Area tier and its replacement by statutory District Health Authorities (DHAs) (DHSS and Welsh Office 1979 p. 9), the retention of FPCs (p. 14), and (somewhat tentatively) the abolition of CHCs (p. 14). The proposals were therefore more than a little different from those of the Royal Commission. Other proposals in Patients First were the simplification of the planning system (p. 18) and greater delegation of authority to 'units' (levels of organisation such as hospitals, below the District) which would be managed by an administrator, and a nurse 'of appropriate seniority to discharge an individual responsibility in conjunction with the medical staff' (p. 7); the administrator at hospital level, rather than a District specialist was to be responsible for functions such as catering and domestic work. The desirability of a 'chief executive' was explicitly rejected (p. 7),though it was suggested that Consultants' contracts of employment be uniformly held by DHAs (p. 11). Experimentation with 'management advisory services' wthin Regions was also announced (pp. 18-19). A later announcement accepted the Royal Commision's critique of NHS information provision and established an investigation under Mrs Edith Korner (DHSS 1980a).

Most of the proposed changes were subsequently brought into operation. With effect from April 1982 DHAs were created, often, though not invariably, on the basis of the former Districts; as a result, FPCs often covered more than one new DHA. At District level consensus DMTs were retained, whilst the Unit level administrator and nurse were to manage in conjunction with a representative of medical staff (DHSS 1980b, para 26) in a triumvirate along the lines originally legitimised in the Bradbeer Report (see above). Special emphasis was placed on the co-ordinating role of the administrator (DHSS 1980b para. 25). CHCs were retained in existence and Consultant contracts were not devolved (DHSS 1981a). The 1982 structure is summarised in Figure 2.3. Parallel changes occurred in Wales (DHSS and Welsh Office 1979 pp. 21-22) and Scotland (Levitt and Wall 1984 pp. 78-101) where the new Authorities were mainly based on the former Areas rather than Districts.

BEHIND THE FORMALITIES

From this long history of developing management and organisation in the NHS three salient observations can be made. These were summarised at the beginning of this Chapter, and each is now discussed in turn.

Lack of Managerial Control of Doctors
In the period from 1948 to about 1982, governments have had little real interest in control of doctors by NHS managers. This can be illustrated in two ways. Firstly, the position of doctors throughout the various formal changes can be examined. The position of GPs has not merely remained constant since the inception of the NHS in 1948, but since the introduction of 'panel doctors' in 1912; the insistence upon remaining as independent contractors and upon precluding even a salary option led to the substitution of Executive Councils for the old Local Insurance Committees. As Willcocks (1967 p. 74) expressed it 'this old compromise was to be the new compromise'. The compromise was again maintained through FPCs in 1974 and 1982 reorganisations, with apparently little attempt to propose alternatives (see, for instance, Medical Services Review Committee 1962 pp. 56, 88-92; DHSS 1970 p. 19), except in the case of the Royal Commission discussed above. In short, there has been little management involvement with general practice; perhaps the significant exception has been the system of prescribing review by which GPs with exceptionally expensive prescribing habits have been identified and asked to modify their practice. (For a graphic account of this system, which can be backed by financial penalties, see Johnson 1962 pp. 51-55).

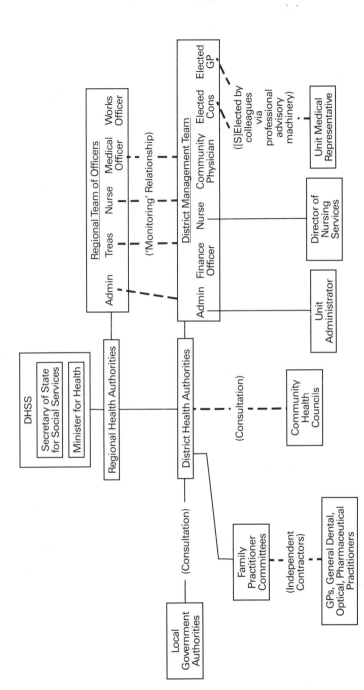

Figure 2.3 Outline Organisation Structure of English NHS: 1982

In summary, it is hardly surprising that both the
Porritt Report and academic commentators noted the
lack of friction between managers and GPs (Medical
Services Review Committee 1962 p. 112; Lindsey 1962
pp. 83-85). Although the 1974 reorganisation
affected the position of MOsH as effectively chief
executives of local authority health departments,
their status was preserved (and in the case of some
of their former subordinates, enhanced) by the
creation of the specialty of Community Medicine.
(See Lewis 1986 for a history of the specialty and
its antecedents).

In hospital medicine too, doctors have not been
challenged by the formal organisation, which,
despite the recommendations of Farquharson-Lang and
the (then) Institute of Hospital Administrators (see
above) remained collegial in character throughout
the period under examination. The clearest
manifestation of this was the creation in 1974 of
consensus teams: a means of providing the formal
right of veto to a group which possessed it in
practice anyway (Harrison 1982 pp. 379-380).
Although the post-1974 Health Authorities had a
smaller medical membership than their predecessors,
this was more than compensated by the formal
involvement of doctors elsewhere in the management
structure. It is significant that consultant
contracts of employment remained at RHA level,
(except in the case of Authorities responsible for
undergraduate medical education), and that no
attempt to introduce American models of hospital
management by clinical 'chiefs of service' was made.
(This was considered and rejected by the Bradbeer
Report: Central Health Services Council, 1954 pp.
27-30). Moreover, the right to engage in private
practice, a major source of uncertainty for
managers, has been retained, and indeed was enhanced
in 1980 (British Medical Journal, 15 September 1979,
p. 685).

A second way of illustrating the adherence of
successive governments to the notion of clinical
freedom is to examine the content of official policy
documents; at all periods in the history of the NHS
such documents have made explicit references either
to the notion itself, or to a model of management
which, it is made clear, centres upon providing
facilities for professionals. Such references
indeed predate the creation of the Service; the 1944
Coalition government White Paper on a National

Health Service stated that 'whatever the organisation, the doctors taking part must remain free to direct their clinical knowledge and personal skill for the benefit of their patients in the way in which they feel to be best' (Ministry of Health 1944 p. 26). These sentiments were on several occasions echoed by Aneurin Bevan, Minister of Health from 1945 to 1951: (see quotations in Allsop 1984 p. 17 and Watkin 1975 p. 139). If such a view underpinned the creation of the NHS, it also underpinned its first reorganisation; the Crossman Green Paper (see above) set out a fundamental principle that 'the Service should provide full clinical freedom to the doctors working in it' (DHSS 1970 p.; see also Allsop 1984 p. 29). The Secretary of State's foreword to the Conservative White Paper which set out the firm plans for Reorganisation assured the reader that

> The organisational changes will not affect the professional relationship between individual patients and individual professional workers on which the complex of health services is so largely built. The professional workers will retain their clinical freedom - governed as it is by the bounds of professional knowledge and ethics and by the resources that are available - to do as they think best for their patients. This freedom is cherished by the professions and accepted by the Government. It is a safeguard for patients today and an insurance for future improvements (DHSS 1972a, p. vii).

The subsequent Grey Book (see above) went further in linking management to medicine:

> ....the objective in reorganising the NHS is to enable health care to be improved. Success in achieving this objective depends primarily on the people in the health care professions who prevent, diagnose and treat disease. Management plays only a subsidiary part, but the way in which the Sevice is organised and the processes used in directing resources can help or hinder the people who play the primary part (DHSS 1972b p. 9).

Nor had the philosophy for what was to become the 1982 reorganisation changed much; Patients First had the following to say:

It is doctors, dentists and nurses and their
colleagues in the other health professions who
provide the care and cure of patients and
promote the health of the people. It is the
purpose of management to support them in giving
that service (DHSS and Welsh Office 1979
pp. 1-2).

Such quotations are, of course, selective. The same
documents also make references to such matters as
the need for efficiency, but what is striking is
that they are careful never to imply that doctors
might need to become more efficient; the inference
is rather that it is other, unspecified, groups
which need to be controlled in order to maximise
resources for medical care. Thus the above
quotation from Patients First continues: 'The
efficient management of the Service is therefore of
the highest importance, not least when resources are
tight. The more economical it can be, the more
resources there will be for patient care' (DHSS and
Welsh Office 1979 p. 3). It is also true that some
of the above documents acknowledge that resources
are limited and that priorities need to be
established. But here again, there is no challenge
to medical autonomy; rather, it is assumed that
agreed priorities will somehow emerge from
discussions. Thus the Grey Book speaks of
mechanisms by which doctors can 'contribute more
effectively to.... decisionmaking' (DHSS 1972b p.
10), whilst Patients First refers to machinery 'to
ensure that the doctor's voice is fully heard' (DHSS
and Welsh Office 1979 p. 17).

In summary, there is little, if any, evidence to
support the view that a desire to increase
managerial control over doctors was the foundation
of changes in NHS organisation and management over
the period under review. Moreover, there is
evidence that NHS managers and interested academics
were themselves perfectly well aware of this, and
did not, as Haywood and Alaszewski (1980 p. 87)
imply, subscribe to the false assumption that they
had a decisive voice in controlling the Service.
Empirical evidence of this is set out Chapter 3; for
the present it can be noted that such influential
figures as Naylor (a Regional Administrator) and
Jaques (a founder of the Brunel approach) agreed
that 'it is not possible to have a "managing
director" ....clinical doctors could not be made
subordinate.....' (Naylor 1971, p 33) Writing of

the same possibility, Jaques (1978 p. 141) later
wrote 'no such solution is realistically
available.'

Better Inputs to Management

The 1960s and 1970s were characterised by a general
belief in the efficacy of organisation structure and
management training as a means of producing better
management in the public sector. Indeed the
recommendations of the Fulton Committee (Committee
on the Civil Service 1968) were based on just these
assumptions. The prevalence of what Klein (1983 p.
90) has termed 'organisational fixes' extended to
the NHS, as the above account has shown; better
management career structures were seen as the answer
to the problem, almost irrespective of what the
problem was. Indeed, in the extreme case the
absence of managerial careers was seen as the
problem; the Salmon Report took it as axiomatic that
nurses' status was too low, and all its proposals
flowed from this (Ministry of Health and Scottish
Home and Health Department 1966 p. 7). Increasing
managerial specialisation (see above) was another
manifestation of the same assumption, as was the
increased attention paid to training and education
of managers (see, for instance, King's Fund Working
Party 1977).

Claims for managerial roles and equality of status
with administrators therefore became the strategy by
which the health professions other than medicine
sought to advance themselves;

> each professional group - which was of course
> heavily represented on the working party
> concerned with its particular specialty - was
> naturally ready to welcome a form of
> organisation which provided more numerous and
> more lucrative opportunities of promotion for
> its members (Watkin 1975 p. 349).

Both the Royal Commission (1979 p. 29) and, more
critically, Brown (1979 p. 31) agreed that consensus
management teams were both a reflection and a cause
of such professional aspirations to managerial
autonomy.

Of course, these claims did not go entirely without
challenge; the content of the Farquharson-Lang and
Institute of Hospital Administrators Reports has
already been discussed. But as the 1974

reorganisation approached, such formal opposition became more muted and disappeared. Its last vestige may be found in Naylor's influential study of the possible forms of new organisation; having dismissed the possibility of management control over clinicians, he continues:

> ....could the remainder of the health professions and all the other groups of workers be subordinated to one director? ....the answer is probably in the affirmative [though] ....as the strength of the other health professions grows nearer to the doctors, there may be pressure for equality of status (Naylor 1971 p. 33).

As is shown in the next Chapter, the status claims of the other professions left some discontent amongst working administrators and doctors; not everyone subscribed to the formal position.

The aspirations of occupational groups thus go a long way towards explaining the changes in NHS organisation and management which occurred between 1948 and the early 1980s. Other factors no doubt contributed; for instance, greater professional and management specialisation were made possible by the construction of larger acute hospitals (Harrison 1981a pp. 38-39). These changes were in turn made possible by professional decisions about the way in which developing medical technology should be exploited (Allen 1979 pp. 52-53; Klein 1983 pp. 74-75). Hence there was an iterative relationship between these factors. It should also be added that the late 1960s and the 1970s were a period in which the co-ordination of welfare state agencies was seen as paramount (see, for instance, Central Policy Review Staff 1975), a view which can be seen in the form adopted in the 1974 reorganisation in particular.

Consumer Protection
It has been seen that a number of institutions related to the interests of the health care consumer were developed in the 1960s and 1970s. These developments cannot however be seen as the product of a conscious concern for consumer views or as a deliberate political or managerial decision to give greater priority to such views. Rather, they were ad hoc reactions to particular problems. The Health Advisory Service and the Health 'Ombudsman' were

28

responses to particular examples of what became a whole series of scandals about the treatment of the inmates of long-stay institutions (Watkin 1978 pp. 72-83). Reforms in the procedure for dealing with hospital complaints also derive from these events (Watkin 1975 p. 208). The creation of CHCs also came about almost accidentally. Klein and Lewis (1976 pp. 11-15) describe how, in the preparations for the 1974 reorganisation, the Conservative Government's emphasis on the managerial role of the members of the new health authorities left a vacuum for a community representative role. They quote one of the Ministers involved as saying 'The idea [of CHCs] suggested itself as soon as we had decided to go for unrepresentative Area Health Authorities' (p. 13).

Developments in consumerism have thus been both reactive and, through the membership of CHCs (see above), directed at the least prestigious part of the NHS. In comparison with other organisational developments, they have been peripheral.

Chapter 3

1948 - 1982: THE MANAGER AS DIPLOMAT

Chapter 2 has examined the formalities of NHS management, but behaviour in organisations is shaped by factors other than the formal roles and structures which have, by and large, been the stuff of NHS reform. This Chapter, by contrast, reviews such empirical research findings as are available concerning the reality of NHS management behaviour in the decade or so prior to the Griffiths Report. The analysis shows substantial consonance between form (as set out in Chapter 2) and substance; the pre-Griffiths NHS manager both was, and was supposed to be, a diplomat rather than a manager of the kind portrayed in the textbooks. He or she was concerned not to procure major change in the shape of health services, but rather to minimise internal conflict and to facilitate the work of health care professionals.

The present Chapter, then, focusses upon a summary of the findings of empirical research into the management of the NHS in the period up to 1982. If studies of the roles of CHCs and of Health Authority (HA) Members are included, the number of projects runs to more than twenty, although some gave rise to more than one publication. The reports of two formal committees of inquiry have also been included. The scope, scale and methods of the studies are summarised in Table 3.1. The list is not, of course, exhaustive, but does include the bulk of relevant research. The Table is ordered in accordance with the commencement date of the fieldwork.

Three observations may be made about these studies. Firstly, it is clear that interest in empirical research in the NHS began to develop in earnest only during the preparatory period for the 1974 reorganisation. Hunter (1986 p. 25) notes, however, that such studies have rarely informed subsequent development in organisation and management, which have tended to have more pragmatic origins. Nor is there evidence to suggest that the phenomena observed are the result of the 1974 reorganisation; the few studies conducted beforehand produced results which are consistent with later studies. Indeed, the middle manager respondents to one post-1974 study were of the opinion that the reorganisation had made no difference (Brown et al 1975 p. 71). Secondly, although a few of the projects produced examples of minority divergent behaviour (these are discussed below), the results of all the research are highly consonant. Thirdly, it should be noted that all the studies are focussed upon relatively senior levels of management; there are no studies of, for instance, managerial behaviour within individual hospital departments. Given that, as Table 3.1 shows, a wide variety of methodology and focus was employed, in projects of varying depth and breadth, there are grounds for confidence in concluding that these findings represent a realistic picture of management in the NHS up to about 1982.

The findings are presented below in the form of four major propositions:

. managers were not the most influential actors in the NHS ('pluralism');
. managerial behaviour was problem-driven rather than objective-driven, in character ('reactiveness');
. managers were reluctant to question the value of existing patterns of service or to propose major changes in them ('incrementalism'); and
. managers behaved 'as if' other groups of employees, rather than the public, were the clients of the NHS ('introversion').

It will be noted that each proposition is in some sense an inversion of a characteristic of the 'textbook' manager, who, it is supposed, pursues organisational objectives related to serving the consumer, via a managerial hierarchy of authority, whilst consistently monitoring the outcomes of decisions (for a selection of classic statements, see Stewart 1979 pp. 66-67). Each proposition is treated below in a separate subsection; in each case the nature of the proposition itself is first elaborated, and the research findings which support the proposition are then outlined.

Table 3.1 Empirical Research in the NHS: 1948-83

AUTHOR(S) AND PUBLICATION DATE	FIELDWORK	SCALE AND SCOPE	METHODS AND SOURCES
FORSYTH (1966)	1964	One RHB & its HMCs	Questionnaire, documents
ROWBOTTOM et al (1973)	1966-72	One RHB & 9 HMCs	Interviews, action research
COMMITTEE OF ENQUIRY INTO ELY HOSPITAL (1969)	1967-68	One hospital	Formal inquiry
BROWN (1979) BROWN et al (1975) HAYWOOD (1977)	1972-75	One Area Health Authority and its predecessors	Interviews, questionnaires, documents, observation
KLEIN & LEWIS (1976)	1974-75	205 CHCs	Questionnaire
HUNTER (1979, 1980, 1984)	1975-77	12 Scottish Health Boards	Questionnaire, interviews, documents, observation in 2 Boards
HAM (1981)	1975-77 (re 1948/74)	One RHB	Documents, interviews
HALLAS (1976)	1975-76	17 CHCs, 60 CHC secretaries	Action research

Table 3.1 Empirical Research in the NHS: 1948-83 (cont'd)

AUTHOR(S) AND PUBLICATION DATE	FIELDWORK	SCALE AND SCOPE	METHODS AND SOURCES
HAYWOOD et al (1979) HAYWOOD (1979) ELCOCK & HAYWOOD (1980) HAYWOOD & ALASZEWSKI (1980)	1975-78	DHSS, 2 RHAS, 4 AHAs and associated Teams	Documents, interviews, observation
BARNARD et al (1979, 1980) LEE & MILLS (1982)	1976-79	2 Area Health Authorities	Documents, interviews, observation
WISEMAN (1979)	1976-78	SHHD, Planning Council, One Scottish Hlth Brd	Documents, interviews, observation
KOGAN et al (1978)	1977	DHSS, Welsh Office, SHHD, 3 RHAs, 6 Area Authorities 8 Districts, 6 CHCs (in England, Wales, Scotland & N Ireland)	Interviews

Table 3.1   Empirical Research in the NHS: 1948-83 (cont'd)

AUTHOR(S) AND PUBLICATION DATE	FIELDWORK	SCALE AND SCOPE	METHODS AND SOURCES
COMMITTEE OF INQUIRY INTO NORMANSFIELD HOSPITAL (1978)	1978	One hospitals	Formal inquiry
HARRISON (1988a) BARNARD & HARRISON (1986)	1978-82	Health Authorities in England	Interviews, questionnaires documents
STEWART et al (1980)	1979	32 District Administrators, 9 Area Administrators	Interviews, observation
HARRISON (1981b)	1979-80	DHSS, professional associations	Interviews, documents
HARDY (1986)	1979-80	2 hospital closures	Interviews, documents
STOCKING (1985)	1980-83	22 innovations in general: 4 detailed cases in RHAs and 12 Districts	Interviews, documents questionnaires
RATHWELL (1987)	1980-84	One HA	Interviews, documents

Table 3.1   Empirical Research in the NHS: 1948-83 (cont'd)

AUTHOR(S) AND PUBLICATION DATE	FIELDWORK	SCALE AND SCOPE	METHODS AND SOURCES
GLENNERSTER et al (1983)	1980-81	2 DHAs, 2 Local Authorities, London	Interviews
SCHULZ & HARRISON (1983)	1981	19 Management Teams	Interviews, documents, some observation
HAM (1986)	1981-85	2 DHAs	Action research
HARRISON et al (1984a)	1982	72 managers	Open ended questionnaire
THOMPSON (1986)	1982-84	7 Management Teams	Interviews, documents
HAYWOOD (1983) HAYWOOD & RANADE (1985)	1982-84	6 DHAs (Members)	Documents, interviews, observation, repertory grid
FORTE (1986)	1983-84	1 District	Documents, interviews

PLURALISM

The term 'pluralism' has been used in political science and related fields, such as industrial relations, to denote a situation where it is alleged that no single actor has dominant influence (see, for instance, Polsby 1980; Fox 1966). The usage of the term here, however, is less specific; it simply means 'not unitary'. Organisation structures are customarily portrayed in a 'family tree' type of diagram, which purports to show a hierarchy of authority flowing from one source (hence 'unitary') at the top; the proposition that the NHS is pluralistic asserts that the Service cannot realistically be represented in such a fashion. In practice, the proposition implies that NHS managers (including DHSS, and HA members) were not the most influential actors; doctors, essentially at local level but to, some extent also as a profession at national level, were the most influential actors. This is, of course, not to argue that either doctors or managers were always unified, or that doctors always got their way. The fact that the NHS functioned like this for so long should not be surprising, since it started life in the same way. All the academic studies of the creation of the NHS (Lindsey 1962; Eckstein 1960; Willcocks 1967) stress the politics of pressure groups and in particular the influence of the medical profession, and it may be considered wishful thinking that a group so powerful at the Service's inception should thereafter eschew influencing its operation.

Management within a health authority is nominally headed by the Chairperson and members of the authority, and since the 1974 reorganisation such persons have had no responsibility for consumer representation, being selected for their personal qualities in a managerial role. Empirical studies of this role have, however, ascribed very little influence to them. Thus Brown et al (1975 pp. 11-14) found that managers gave the authority members very little information about ongoing issues about which there were disagreements. Haywood's initial study of six DHAs concluded that 'in general, there were few decisions influenced by members' (Haywood 1983 p. 44), a finding confirmed in a follow-up study which also indicated that, within HA membership, chairpersons were relatively influential (Haywood and Ranade 1985). These findings have been confirmed by Ham; the general lack of member

influence on policy was partly the result of medical
influence manifest through 'creeping development in
acute specialties' (1986 pp. 123-126). Scottish
members similarly lacked influence on resource
allocation (Hunter 1980 p. 198); one respondent
perhaps summed it all up when he said 'as far as I
can see, the health board is a rubber stamp' (Hunter
1984 p. 50). Managers interviewed by Glennerster et
al (1983 p. 261) and Schulz and Harrison (1983 p.30)
confirmed these assessments of member weakness.

If members were not the most influential actors
within health authorities, neither were managers. A
number of case studies have instanced the influence
of hospital Consultants on specific decisions.
Kogan's research for the Royal Commission on the NHS
documented the case of a decision to transfer the
responsibility for biomedical engineering to the
Works Officer, twice overturned as a result of
medical objections (Kogan et al 1978 p. 129 ff).
This ability to veto change was capable of
persisting over long periods; Rathwell has shown
how, in one health authority, attempts to settle the
number and distribution of hospital beds for the
elderly remained unsuccessful, as a result of
medical disagreements, over a period of four years.
Even a severe winter, and consequent admissions
crisis did not aid resolution, which had still not
been achieved at the conclusion of the research
(1987, Chap 4). In another study, Linstead has
shown how Consultant physicians, on this occasion in
alliance with another professional group, were able
to veto proposed changes in training arrangements
for hospital technicians (1984 p. 11). A further
example of the obstructive ability of the medical
profession is provided in Forte's (1986 p. 43) case
study of one disrict; clinicians were able to delay
the implementation of the whole operational plan by
withdrawing their earlier agreement to acute service
'rationalisations'. The ability of doctors to
impose their definition of a particular situation
upon others has been well illustrated by Ham's
example of proposed alterations to bed allocations
between hospitals being seen as a lack of suitable
case material for medical teaching rather than as a
need to provide a good service for the elderly (Ham
1981 pp. 147-149).

Perhaps more important than such single instances
are findings which show the influence of the medical
profession on the strategic shape of services

delivered by the NHS. Haywood and Alaszewski (1980 pp. 104-106) have examined the pattern of inputs to, and outputs from, the NHS during the 1970s, showing that whilst real resources available (staff, money) rose considerably, output in terms of the number of cases treated (as inpatients or outpatients) rose much more modestly. Although this discrepancy is to some extent due to improvements in staff conditions of employment, the major explanation is increased intensity of diagnosis and treatment, a conclusion confirmed by increases in the workload of pathology, radiology and physiotherapy departments, and by the rising ratio of total attendances to new outpatients. Some of this pattern is illustrated by figure 3.1, which can be seen as implying a decision, not taken by politicians or managers but by individual clinicians, to devote the majority of additional resources to greater intensity of care rather than to treating larger numbers of patients. That is, the decisions which underlie these aggregates are individual clinicians' decisions about admission, diagnosis, therapy, and discharge. (It should be appreciated, of course, that these conclusions involve no judgement about the value or otherwise of such trends.) These observations, together with an analysis of failures to implement national priorities, also led the authors to comment that 'the power of [central government] to effect change is limited, even when only a modest change in emphasis is envisaged' (p. 61), a conclusion supported in Stocking's study of the pattern of introduction of day case surgery (1985 pp. 223-228).

This strategic influence of the medical profession can also be discerned in the arrangements for the education and supply of professional manpower, a crucial resource for the NHS. Harrison's study of this area concluded that the arrangements were to varying degrees dominated by professional organisations rather than by managers or even by DHSS. Underneath a complex surface pattern of many official and professional bodies was, however, a dominant medical influence; 'the whole mechanism is not nearly as [plural] as the mere listing of the bodies involved may convey; not only is the medical profession dominant within most of them, but the same sections of the profession ... are represented within many' (Harrison 1981b p. 94). Kogan et al (1978 p. 174) have pointed out that decisions by bodies such as the General Medical Council can result in the non-recognition of hospital training

Figure 3.1   Some Hospital Statistics, England, 1971-1977

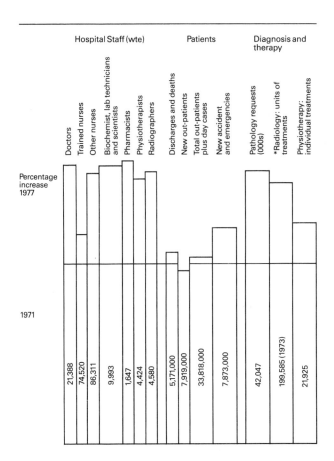

Source: S. Haywood and A. Alaszewski, *Crisis in the Health Service: the Politics of Management,* Croom Helm 1980. Reproduced by permission.

posts which in turn can result in hospital closure.

Conclusions about strategic medical influence are also supported by research into the management and policy process in specific NHS Regions. Elcock and Haywood (1980 pp. 77, 97) note that 'in both Regions, the medical profession fought vigorously against changes in priorities intended to favour the [official priority groups of patients] at the expense of the acute sector.' Nor do such conclusions relate solely to the post-reorganisation period. Ham's historical study concluded that legal and financial controls were not an effective means of securing change; 'the capacity of the central [government] department to ensure that its policies were implemented was limited' even though 'its style became more promotional and interventionist as the 1960s progressed' (Ham 1981 pp. 191-192). Stocking's 1985 study of such longstanding central priorities as Regional Secure Units and the revision of waking times for hospital inpatients confirms this conclusion.

How far are such conclusions supported by evidence about the perceptions of NHS managers? In an interview study of eighteen management teams, Schulz and Harrison found that

> on twelve.... teams.... there was overwhelming agreement that consultants had the primary influence on the pattern of health care delivery in the area. Only two teams ascribed the primary influence to themselves, with the remaining four.... either divided on the issue or ascribing equal influence' (Schulz and Harrison 1983 p. 33).

The same respondents reported that RHAs and DHSS were relatively uninfluential (pp. 30-33). These perceptions were replicated in another interview study of administrators, medical and nursing officers, who were 'particularly aware of the power consultants had to cause and prevent change. They saw the individual professional largely in control' (Glennerster et al 1983 p. 260).

Nor were the managers themselves unified; 'what was striking was the extent to which most participants agreed about what they actually saw happening in.... inter departmental behaviour: it was very close to a bureaucratic politics model most of the time' (Glennerster et al, 1983, p. 263). Thompson's more recent study of teams has shown a high level of bargaining between DMT members, without the formation of stable coalitions (1986 pp. 29, 34, 54-56). A general suspicion of colleagues at organisational levels other than the respondent's own has surfaced in other studies (see, for instance, Stewart et al 1980 p. 66; Haywood et al 1979 pp. 26, 35), as has a degree of discontentment with the organisational arrangements created in 1974. Haywood et al (1979 p. 39) report a tendency for chief administrators and medical officers to perceive a relative loss of power, a finding reflected in Schulz and Harrison's respondents' perceptions of consensus decisionmaking (1983, Table 1), and the observation that 'many team members of all categories [state] that they would ideally prefer a chief executive officer arrangement if they could be the chief executive' (p. 17). A survey on behalf of the chief administrators' pressure group indicated a good deal of discontent with consensus decisionmaking, especially on the part of Area Administrators (Fairey et al (1975 pp. 25-26), a view shared by the District Administrators in Stewart's study (Stewart et al 1980 pp. 30, 113, 117-118). Other studies (see, for instance, Kogan et al 1978 pp. 45 ff) have demonstrated a much greater level of approval of the 1974 team arrangements, apparently on a pragmatic basis; this is further discussed in the conclusion to this Chapter.

The overall conclusion to be drawn from the research is that doctors were the most powerful group in the NHS: small wonder that as a profession they were broadly content with the Service's management arrangements. Forsyth's study showed that consultants were happy with an administration which was 'reluctant to exert authority' (1966 pp. 128-130), even to the extent of preferring the Porritt proposals for administrative unification of the Service (see above) to the argument of the contemporary Gillie Report that the NHS should be co-ordinated through the activities of GPs. It has already been noted that GPs' evidence to the Porritt Committee indicated their contentment with the arrangements. Unfortunately, there has been relatively little recent research aimed at eliciting the perceptions of rank-and-file consultants, though research into perceptions of clinical freedom by Harrison et al (1984b) did indicate a continuing support for the principle of consensus teams.

Two further observations can be made from the body of research which is being discussed; the first concerns the management arrangements originally created in 1974. It has already been noted that the system of consensus decisionmaking was to some extent a recognition of the pre-existing influence of doctors; organisational features such as the election of clinicians to teams and elaborate professional advisory machinery can be seen as an attempt to manage this situation. Research shows that, as such, they met with only limited success. Hence influence attributed to elected clinical team members did not even approximate to that attributed to consultants at large (Schulz and Harrison 1983 pp. 26-27), whilst professional advisory machinery was ineffective because individual doctors were unwilling to surrender their own power to it (Brown et al 1975 pp 16, 50-51; Brown 1979 p. 138). Consensus decisionmaking, rather than, as intended, allowing controversial issues to pass for resolution to the health authority (DHSS 1972b p. 30), resulted in such issues being suppressed (Kogan et al 1978 p. 47) and 'the avoidance of solutions which might threaten personal relationships between team members' (Haywood 1977 p. 28).

The second and final observation is that, once doctors are disregarded, managers, or more precisely, administrators, are seen as the most influential amongst the remaining actors. Thus Stewart et al (1980 pp. 35, 81, 83) rated District Administrators as highly influential, partly because of their access to information. Similarly, Schulz and Harrison (1983 p. 24) show that top. managers regarded the chief administrator as the most powerful actor, other than hospital consultants, in the resource allocation process. The relative lack of influence of trade unions, at least when confronted by managers competent in political skills, has been shown in Hardy's (1986 p. 11) study of hospital closure and Harrison's (1988a) study of demands for union membership. agreements. The lack of influence of HA members has already been mentioned.

REACTIVENESS

Just as the notion of pluralism contrasts with the textbook model of managerial authority, tho notion

of reactiveness in managerial behaviour contrasts
with the textbook view of proactive, goal-seeking
behaviour: establishing objectives and then
initiating action on the part of others to ensure
that these are met. In practice however, this
distinction is likely to be one of degree rather
than absolute; Larson et al (1986 p. 388 ff) have
pointed out the difficulties in applying the
distinction to observations of managerial behaviour,
and studies of top managers in industries other than
the NHS have shown that executive work is much more
fragmented and problem-oriented than the textbook
picture suggests (Kotter 1982 p. 79 ff; Mintzberg
1973 p. 31 ff). The sense in which 'reactiveness'
is employed here denotes that NHS managers (unlike,
for instance, the general managers in Kotter's
research) had problems brought to them or thrust
upon them, rather than themselves seeking problems
or setting objectives.

The process of planning is where, perhaps, one might
most expect to find proactive behaviour; studies of
NHS planning show that this was rarely possible.
For instance, Barnard et al (1979, Vol 3, p. 16)
document the way in which a London health
authority's attempts to assess the health care needs
of its population were rapidly abandoned in order to
produce 'defensive' information to demonstrate the
perceived unfairness to the authority of the RAWP
formula. The northern health district studied by
Forte (1986 pp. 24-25) experienced similar
difficulty in sustaining proactive behaviour. In
Scotland, Hunter found '... plans thwarted by
the flare-up of a crisis, such as occurred in
both [health boards where fieldwork was conducted]
over nuring staff establishments' (1980 p. 151),
whilst even within the Scottish Home and Health
Department planning was reactive and ad hoc (Wiseman
1979 pp. 106-107).

It might also be expected that proactive behaviour
would be found in the activities of chief officers
of health authorities, and the management teams of
which they were members. In their study of District
Administrators, Stewart et al (1980 p. 76) note,
however, that few were able to play the more
proactive roles of shaping plans, innovating new
practices or of managing the total organisation;
rather the evidence (pp. 149-171) of how the
research subjects spent their days shows little
sign of interest in strategic issues but a

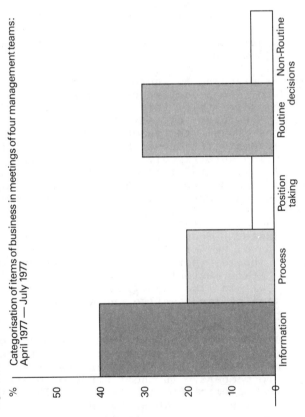

Figure 3.2 A Sample of Management Team Agenda Items

% Categorisation of items of business in meetings of four management teams: April 1977 — July 1977

Information   Process   Position taking   Routine decisions   Non-Routine decisions

* 100% = 671 items of business

Source: S. Haywood, 'Team Management in the NHS: What is it All About', *Health and Social Service Journal*, 5 October 1979.

preoccupation with ad hoc referrals of issues. Nor was the content of management team agendas any different; Schulz and Harrison (1983 p. 37) note that a major item of team work was 'tackling of issues which in some way presented themselves as problems to the team or its members'. Haywood's systematic classification of the agenda items of several management teams shows the prevalance of non-strategic items (Haywood 1979 pp. 54, 57). Figure 3.2 summarises these findings; 90% of items consist of information exchange, deciding to whom issues should be referred ('process'), or routine decison-making. Yet the teams were created in order to take 'decisions for the totality of health care' (DHSS 1972b p. 15). Haywood summarises by describing chief officers as 'directors of process.... reactors rather than initiators....' (1979 p. 59).

If top managers were reactive, it is hardly .urprising that their subordinates perceived their own jobs in the same way. Harrison, Haywood and Fussell took a population of upper-middle NHS managers all attending university continuing education courses (and perhaps therefore to be expected to be more textbook-oriented than the average) and gave them a free choice of how to make a written characterisation of their own job roles. The respondents overwhelmingly chose to typify their jobs as tackling problems referred to them by other actors who had expressed some dissatisfaction; the main consideration was to satisfy the complaint without creating further dissatisfactions elsewhere (Harrison et al 1984a p. 186).

It is not necessarily the case that such departures from the textbook management model constitute grounds for criticism, and indeed the thrust of the present Chapter is to argue that the behaviour of NHS managers in the period under consideration in fact reflected what was expected of them. In extreme circumstances, however, such behaviour can become an appropriate target for censure. The Normansfield Report, for instance, provides an example of management passivity and reluctance to act against a consultant member of medical staff which led eventually to a major scandal over the treatment of patients (Committee of Inquiry 1978 p. 386 ff; also Klein 1978 p. 1803).

Drawing on their pre-reorganisation reseach, Rowbottom et al concluded that 'Administrators were

the co-ordinators, the middle-men [sic], the fixers
....the exact nature of their authority was
uncertain the extreme' (1973 p. 172). The evidence
suggests that after 1974 this conclusion was equally
applicable to NHS managers generally.

INCREMENTALISM

The notion of incrementalism was first systematically theorised by Lindblom (1959), who
subsequently distinguished between incremental
change, that is, change taking place in small steps,
incremental analysis, that is, an approach to
decisionmaking which severely limits the number and
nature of the alternatives considered and 'partisan
mutual adjustment', a process of interaction where
actions of participants affect actions of others,
producing outcomes which differ from the intentions
of any actor (Lindblom 1979 pp. 517-522). One
obvious problem in labelling particular changes as
'incremental' is that it is a matter of judgement as
to what represents a small step; in any case, a
number of successive small steps can quickly add up
to a major change (Etzioni 1967 p. 386). For
present purposes, however, this problem can be
avoided by looking at incremental analysis:

> Simplification is systematically achieved in
> two principal ways.... it is achieved through
> limitation of policy comparisons to those which
> differ in relatively small degree from policies
> presently in effect.... [and] it is necessary
> only to study those respects in which the
> proposed alternative and its consequences
> differ from the status quo (Lindblom 1959 p.
> 84).

In other words the status quo is largely taken for
granted and not subjected to any review or evaluation. To the extent that policy change is at all
attributed to managers, therefore, it can be deduced
that 'simple incremental analysis' (Lindblom 1979 p.
517) on their part will serve to reinforce the
status quo. It is this lack of critical review of,
and general attention to, the existing pattern of
services which characterised the behaviour of NHS
managers in the period under examination. (It is
argued below that 'partisan mutual adjustment' is
not a good description of relationships between
doctors and managers.)

One way of approaching this is to look at the nature of planning options explored. These show a strong emphasis on hospital beds; thus Rathwell (1987 Chapter 4) has shown how planning for the elderly in one authority was largely confined to beds, notwithstanding the existence of official priority for community care. (In the same study, planning for the mentally handicapped, where no beds existed, was not so constrained.) Similarly Ham (1981 p. 147) has shown how in another city the problems of the elderly were perceived as a problem of 'bed blocking', and Glennerster et al (1983 p. 261) have shown the importance with which national norms were treated. Planning options also showed a strong emphasis on what Brown et al termed 'shopping lists of deficiencies' in existing services:

> When the.... district teams submitted their....
> priorities for long-term development.... over
> half concerned the development of primary care
> .... [but] when it came to concrete
> proposals.... 'community' projects did not fare
> quite so well.... They received.... their
> pre-reorganisation share of the share-out
> (Brown et al 1975 pp. 103-104).

According to Thompson (1986 p. 20), things had not changed by the 1980s. Such ad hoc planning was also to be found in Scotland (Wiseman 1979), though planning documents sometimes sought to conceal this by the inclusion of large quantities of symbolic information unrelated to actual proposals for change (Schulz and Harrison 1983 p. 38). Glennerster et al (1983 p. 264) note that most of the respondents in their study 'still thought of planning as what to do with the increment' and also provide an insight into why this should be so; 'in theory, people favoured a change in priorities but only on the basis of "you can do it so long as you don't touch me"' (p. 260).

A further characteristic of planning options follows closely from this. Hunter (1980 pp. 145, 184) notes that development funds were not merely regarded as important, but for many actors were the answer to planning problems; the tendency was always to seek more resources rather than to question the value of existing resource use, most developments were the result of building schemes, and most also meant 'more of the same'. He goes on to explain:

> At best, allocations of [development funds]

reflected a compromise between.... simply plugging gaps in existing services and.... initiating new services.... Often there was no choice.... Pressures from existing services presented officers with little or no alternative but to plough more funds into them to relieve the pressures (Hunter 1980 p. 184, emphasis added).

The same absence of evaluation or review was prevalent in managerial behaviour more generally. The management teams in Schulz and Harrison's study allocated resources incrementally; when asked individually about their objectives, respondents overwhelmingly replied that they were concerned, firstly, to keep existing services intact, and, secondly, to respond if possible to internal demands for expansion. Movement towards national priorities came only in third place (Schulz and Harrison 1983 p 37). Not surprisingly, therefore, Barnard et al (1979, Vol 3, p. 32) found that 'little attention was paid to collecting information on resource use ....or on outcomes.' To some extent, however, the illusion of scrutiny was maintained by such devices as frequent visits to institutions by senior officers, though these were in practice quite uncritical in approach (Schulz and Harrison 1983 p. 37); there is clearly no necessary connection between critical evaluation and this practice of 'management by wandering about' (Peters and Waterman 1982 p. 121 ff). In a more recent study Thompson (1986 p. 57) was surprised to observe 'the noticeable absence of any systematic monitoring.... of policy formulation and implementation.'

The same approach to management was manifested in Harrison, Haywood and Fussell's study of upper middle managers; respondents were given the opportunity to choose a problem related to their work, and to state how they would tackle it and what would be a satisfactory solution. The tendency was for responses to ignore the last section of the brief, that is to treat the action taken to attack the problem as being a solution in itself, rather than to suggest criteria by which the results of that action might be judged (Harrison et al 1984b p. 186). In the light of this varied evidence, it is difficult to disagree with the conclusion that the managerial changes of the 1970s failed to make NHS decisionmaking less incremental (Brown 1979 p. 205; Lee and Mills 1982 p. 179).

INTROVERSION

The notion of reactiveness (see above) has been defined in terms of managerial behaviour triggered primarily by problems referred to managers by other actors. A natural further question to ask would be what kinds of problem and what other actors? The notion of introversion summarises the answer to this question; both the sources and nature of management problems were to be found inside the organisation, rather than outside it in the form of patients, relatives or public. In other words managerial action was producer-led rather than consumer-led.

Firstly, it can be established that CHCs, the official representatives of the health care consumer, had relatively little impact. Hallas concluded from his research in one Region that:

> On the whole, Councils have been far too polite and deferential.... the tendency [is] to accept information on trust.... to assume that if persons have a string of qualifications and/or resounding titles, then they are to be deferred to, even in matters which are not within their professional competence (Hallas 1976 p. 59).

And CHCs were reluctant to use the modest formal authority that they had been given in 1974:

> With rare exceptions they accepted, without much demur, proposals for closing down hospitals and wards: a pattern which is all the more interesting since this is one of the few areas of activity where CHCs actually have some power, even if it is only the power of delay (Klein and Lewis 1976 p. 135).

These studies occurred in the early days of CHCs, and it is certainly the case that they subsequently became much more active in resisting closures (Allsop 1984 p. 197). However, by the 1980s CHCs were still reporting difficulty over getting acceptance for their notion of 'consultation' (Ham 1980 p. 226), and top managers regarded them as uninfluential (Schulz and Harrison 1983 p. 30-33). Writing of the consultation process of which CHCs were only a part, Lee and Mills concluded (1982 p. 142) that 'few of those [bodies] consulted perceived much benefit to be gained from the formal consultation process.'

Secondly, studies of NHS managers' behaviour show
that their attention was strongly focussed within
the organisation rather than outwards. Stewart et
al (1980 pp. 172-177) traced all issues with which
district administrators dealt over a three-day
period, almost none of which did not originate
within the health authority. Similarly, all the
examples of decisions quoted in Haywood's study
(1979 pp. 57-58) are internal in origin. The Howe
Report into the scandal at Ely hospital (see above
Chapter 2) had shown a closed community with no
awareness of standards elsewhere and an inbuilt
resistance to complaints (Committee of Enquiry 1969
p. 115 ff) (and it was seen that this was not the
first or last such scandal), so that Thompson's
comment from a study conducted in the early 1980s is
apposite:

> One of the more sobering features of the study
> was an apparent lack of interest in consumer
> responses, even the relevance and significance
> of patients' complaints (Thompson 1986 p. 57).

The same kind of introversion is evident in the
responses to the study by Harrison, Haywood and
Fussell. Tables 3.2 and 3.3 show, respectively,
'characteristic' work problems freely chosen by
administrator and nurse manager respondents. In the
case of the administrators agendas are largely
defined by other actors within the health authority,
whilst the nurses' agendas seem dominated by
problems of organisational formalities. The
authors concluded that:

> the ....study suggests ....that the typical
> dissatisfactions which NHS managers perceive as
> problems are related not to formal
> organisational objectives as set out in
> statute, nor.... to the kind.... (such as
> quality, access, acceptability and equality)
> suggested by the Royal Commission on the
> National Health Service, but to organisational
> process and internal relationships.... The
> material counsels against any expectations of
> logical or causal links between formal
> organisational objectives, managers' percep-
> tions, and managerial action (Harrison et al
> 1984a p. 1987).

CONCLUSION: THE MANAGER AS DIPLOMAT

The present chapter has examined the realities of management in the first twenty-odd years of the NHS. The first conclusion from this examination is that they are consonant with the formal position explored in the preceeding Chapter. Managers neither were, nor were supposed to be, influential with respect to doctors. The quality of management (like the quality of the Service itself; Long et al 1985 p. 224) was judged by its inputs. Managers in general worked to solve problems and to maintain their organisations rather than to secure major change. And, at least as far as managers were concerned, the consumer was marginalised. It should also be noted that evidence about how managers behave is highly consistent with evidence about what they say (Harrison 1986; Stewart et al 1980 p. 46).

The four propositions which were used to structure the summary of research findings in the latter half of the Chapter are consistent with each other, and when taken together provide a coherent picture of the NHS manager which can be summed up in one word: diplomat. Keeling's model of the diplomat is a modest one: 'the diplomat's ambition for the day is perhaps to see an advance in the affairs in which he is involved ....hopefully a few less decisions bogged down' (1972 p. 106). Applying the notion of diplomacy to the NHS, Harrison and Hallas defined it thus:

....a process concerned to conciliate, in as co-ordinated a fashion as possible, all the sub-groups within an organisation (Harrison and Hallas 1979a p. 1486).... In the context of diplomacy there is rarely a meaningful overall objective; more often there is a set of par-tially, or sometimes completely, contradictory objectives held by groups or individuals (1979b p. 1523).

Keeling's list of diplomatic skills shows how far such a model of management is from that which is found in the textbook: sensitivity to opportunities for fine adjustment, knowledge of when to work quickly and when slowly, skill in political argument and in negotiations, and flexibility even to the point of reversing goals (Keeling 1972 pp. 106-108).

None of this is to suggest that NHS managers never

Table 3.2   Typical Problems: Group of
             Administrators (1982)

Respondent	Summary of Problem
1	An enquiry from a nursing officer about restrictions on visiting arrangements for a 16-year-old male patient.
2	Change the method of management of porters and drivers and reorganise shift work to increase flexibility.
3	Unwillingness of staff recreation team to allow the league of friends to participate fully in hospital activities, and in particular a reluctance to hand over to them the organisation of the hospital fete.
4	Evening domestics refused cover for the absence of one of their colleagues on maternity leave.
5	New member of consultant staff requests accommodation for an out-patient clinic on a day and time when none is available in hospital.
6	Difference of interpretation of policy about terms of replacement of staff in a period when numbers of "funded" posts were being reduced in the district.
7	Claim for up-grading of post in pathology department.
8	Industrial action by sewing room ladies.
9	Reorganisation of copying facilities in district headquarters to minimise waiting time and obtain correct balance of machines at other locations.
10	Delay in re-opening of post-natal ward during building project.
11	Inappropriate siting of physiotherapy facilities on large site, occasioning treatment in wards not considered to be the "correct environment".
12	Allocation of responsibility between patient sevices officer and voluntary service co-ordinator for newly opened patients club run in the evening by volunteers.

Table 3.2   Typical Problems: Group of
             Administrators (1982) (cont'd)
Respondent   Summary of Problem

13   Visit by health authority during
             "mild" industrial action likely to
             "lead to more severe demonstration".
14   "Messy documentation" for each stage
             of grievance procedure for an
             ambulance service.

Table 3.3   Typical Problems: Group of Nurse Managers
             (1982)
Respondent   Summary of Problem

20   Communication and role patterns in
             nurse education division.
21   Organisational arrangements for
             nursing in a geographically defined
             management unit.
22   Organisational arrangements for
             integration of midwifery with acute
             nursing unit.
23   Development of a model of nurse
             manpower demand and supply.
24   Organisational arrangements within a
             mental illness/geriatrics unit of
             mangement.
25   Recruitment and selection procedure
             for learner nurses at end of training
             period.
26   Relationships with administration in
             a hospital: design of policy for
             relief staffing.
27   Formal incident reporting procedure
             in hospital.

Source: Harrison et al (1984a); reproduced by
permission.

sought to influence doctors or that they were never successful. A few of the studies which were discussed above did provide examples of management behaviour which was more proactive and less incremental than the norm. Unfortunately, these have not been well investigated. Stewart et al (1980 p. 78 ff) imply that some district administrators were able to be proactive, but do not attempt to explain why. Schulz and Harrison (1983 pp. 40-43) note that a few management teams were proactive: they 'fully recognised their general lack of influence, [but] were prepared to look.... for areas where they could carry more weight, and actively to pursue objectives related to health and efficiency.' But beyond noting that such teams often contained a respected medical officer and that the effect seemed to result from synergy, no further explanation is offered. Rathwell's single case study comes closest to providing a plausible explanation; the successful relationship between a joint care planning team, a local authority, and voluntary organisation was possible because it related to mental handicap in an authority where there were no existing beds, and therefore no vested interests at stake (Rathwell 1987, Chaps 4, 8). Managers certainly experience some frustrations too (Klein 1984a p. 1708), and it has been shown that some felt that the 1974 reorganisation diminished their authority. But in general NHS managers were both uninfluential in relation to doctors and reluctant to use what potential influence they had (Schulz and Harrison 1983 p. 39).

As a result, there was little conflict between doctors and managers. No doubt doctors sometimes felt that managers did not fully understand their needs (Medical Services Review Committee 1962 pp. 110-111) but Heller (1979 pp. 1, 45) and Petchey (1986 p. 100) are mistaken in arguing that managers have striven to rationalise the Service and consequently that its shape is a product of their conflicts with the medical profession. Nor is Klein (1985a p. 60) necessarily correct in arguing that doctors and managers have conflicting value systems. On the contrary, and in contrast to local authority social service departments (Kakabadse 1982 p. 109), there has been a remarkable homogeneity of culture in the NHS. Doctors and managers have shared common values (Brown 1979 p. 191), and common hierarchies in terms of the status attached to particular medical specialties and to acute, teaching, hospitals (Schulz and Harrison 1983 p. 44).

Such conflicts as occurred were elsewhere. Industrial relations in the NHS were periodically difficult between 1970 and about 1982, and increasingly militant behaviour by manual workers in particular made managers behave in a more circumspect fashion than before, although the substantive impact of such militancy was slight (Harrison 1988a; Barnard and Harrison 1986) and the origin of much of it was in national pay disputes (Bosanquet 1979).

This situation of medical dominance can be re-stated in the language of Figure 1.2 above. Third-party (government) control over physicians, has been limited to the control of aggregate resource flow. Managers (of all disciplines) have acted as agents for physicians, facilitating their practice by solving problems, smoothing conflicts and generally maintaining the organisation. For the span of time covered by this Chapter managers can, therefore, be classified along with physicians in a passive alliance rather than on active conspiracy. Moreover, despite a major dispute over private hospital beds, almost certainly unintended (Klein 1980), there has been little conflict between government and doctors, the former having been largely concerned to limit total NHS resources, within which doctors have been left free to act as they wished (Klein 1984a p. 1706). The 'partisan mutual adjustment' aspect of incrementalism has not, therefore, been a good general description of the dynamics of NHS politics up to 1982, which can be better characterised in theoretical terms by Dunleavy's notion of 'ideological corporatism':

....the effective integration of different organisations and institutions.... by the acceptance or dominance of an effectively unified view of the world.... [T]he active promotion of changes in ideas rests quite largely with individual professionals.... bargained or negotiated compromises will be relatively rare (pp. 8-9).... the distinction between formulation and implementation may dissolve altogether.... so that policy is just what professionals in the field do (Dunleavy 1981 p. 13).

Chapter 4

1982 - 1984: THE MANAGER AS SCAPEGOAT

As Chapter 3 has shown, the diplomat role of the NHS
manager persisted over a long period, up to 1982 and
perhaps for a year or two beyond (Thompson 1986).
But from 1982 onwards there occurred a series of
central government initiatives in which the
legitimacy of the diplomat role was steadily eroded,
and in which managers were increasingly portrayed as
culpable for the shortcomings of the Service. The
manager's transition to the status of scapegoat did
not take place suddenly; the period under discussion
was one of considerable turbulence for the NHS, in
which the implementation of earlier reform
decisions, such as the abolition of the Area tier
of organisation and experiments with a management
advisory service, occurred alongside the newer
initiatives. These initiatives culminated in a
number of major changes in the management
arrangements for the NHS, stemming from the
Griffiths Report (NHS Management Inquiry 1983).
This Chapter gives an account of these initiatives
and the value-judgements which underlie them. The
conclusion argues that these imply a challenge to
the medical profession: an attempt to shift the
frontier of control between government and doctors
by (in terms of Figure 1.2) detaching managers from
the provider category and converting them into
agents for the third party, the government itself.

THE PRE-GRIFFITHS INITIATIVES

From 1981 onwards the NHS had been expected by the
government to make 'efficiency savings'; this
practice consisted of assuming that health
authorities' outturn expenditure would be less than
their nominal budget by a specified percentage, and
hence providing an actual budget to match only the
assumed outturn. Since such an arrangement provides
no controls over where the savings are made, it is

no more than a convenient assumption that they result from improved efficiency (Harrison and Gretton 1984 p.97). The required figures were 0.2% in 1981-2, 0.3% in 1982-3 and 0.5% in 1983-4 (Ham 1985 p.48).

The announcements made by the then new Secretary of State, Mr Norman Fowler, on 22 January 1982 of arrangements to 'improve accountability' in the NHS (DHSS 1982a) represented something altogether more sophisticated. There were two elements to these arrangements: a review process and a set of performance indicators.

The review process was intended to secure greater adherence to national policies and priorities than had previously been the case (see Chapter 3 above);

.... each year Ministers will lead a Departmental review of the long-term plans, objectives and effectiveness of each Region with the Chairmen of the Regional Authorities and Chief Regional Officers. The aims of the new system will be to ensure that each Region is using the resources allocated to it in accordance with the Government's policies - for example giving priority to services for the elderly, the handicapped and the mentally ill - and also to establish agreement.... on the progress and development which the Regions will aim to achieve in the ensuing year (DHSS 1982a, pp.1-2).

A similar process was to take place between regional authorities and DHAs within the region. The new process, commenced immediately, in January 1982, with a review of the Mersey Region.

Performance Indicators were to be developed on a pilot basis in the Northern Region. To be employed in conjunction with the review process, they would

.... enable comparison to be made between districts and so help Ministers and the Regional Chairmen.... to assess the performance of their constituent.... authorities in using manpower and other resources efficiently. (DHSS 1982a p.2).

Unlike earlier attempts to use comparative data (see, for instance, Yates 1983), the new indicators

were therefore to be compulsory. The first national
(English) package of indicators (DHSS 1983a) was
issued on 22 September 1983, in a form which allowed
any health authority to be compared with all others
in terms both of absolute values of the indicators
used and of rankings within the region and the
country. The package contained some seventy
indicators relating to clinical work, finance,
manpower (sic), support services and estate
management, all constructed from already available
data. The clinical indicators related mainly to the
use of clinical facilities within broad specialty
groups, rather than to the outcomes of treatment,
consisting of such efficiency measures as average
length of hospital stay, throughput of patients per
bed per annum, turnover interval betweeen cases
occupying a bed, and the ratio of return outpatient
visits to new outpatients. They are, however, all
measures which are largely determined by the
aggregate of doctors' behaviour rather than by
managers' decisions.

A number of criticisms of the first package were
made (Pollitt 1985a; Rathwell and Barnard 1985).
Firstly, some indicators were ambiguous in that it
was not clear whether high, or low, values
represented 'good' performance. Secondly, it was
known that many of the original data sources were of
dubious accuracy. Thirdly, the physical format of
indicator presentation in a very thick book of
typescript tables was held to be user-unfriendly.
Finally, the absence of data related to health care
outcome was criticised. A number of joint DHSS/NHS
working groups were established to revise the
indicators, and to extend them beyond hospitals, and
a revised package was issued on 19 July 1985 (DHSS
1985a). The new indicators went some way towards
meeting the first three criticisms (in particular,
by using computer graphics), but still lacked
measures related to the effectiveness of treatment
(Pollitt 1985b). An indicator of medically
preventable deaths was added in 1987; (see Charlton
et al 1983 for the basis of this).

Less than two months after the original review
process/performance indicator announcement, Mr
Fowler announced two further initiatives (DHSS
1982b). Firstly, a national enquiry was established
with the aim of 'identify[ing] underused and surplus
land and property, and, where appropriate
dispos[ing] of it' (p.1). The subsequent Ceri

Davies Report (DHSS 1983b) recommended a system of notional rents for NHS property as the basis of a performance measure of estate utilisation and the disposal of unused and underused assets; it was accepted by the Government in November 1983 (DHSS 1983c). The other initiative was the experimental use of private firms of accountants to audit the accounts of health authorities (DHSS 1982b).

Only three weeks from this announcement, on 1 April 1982, came the announcement of yet another initiative: the extension of 'Rayner Scrutinies' from the Civil Service to the NHS. Named after Sir Derek Rayner, Managing Director of Messrs Marks and Spencer and part-time efficiency adviser to Government, such scrutinies involve intensive study of a particular area of expenditure by an officer seconded from normal duties (DHSS 1982c). The chosen topics were later announced as vacancy advertising, the storage of supplies, catering costs, the cost-effectiveness of meetings, NHS residential property, the recovery of aids loaned to patients, ambulance service control systems, collection of income due to health authorities, and the administration of project briefs for hospital building schemes (DHSS 1982d).

Further initiatives followed. On 27 August a Review of NHS Audit arrangements was announced; the results, promulgated a year later, emphasised the need for greater attention to be given to 'value for money' rather than to narrow financial propriety (DHSS 1982e; 1983d). On 7 October 1982 it was announced that a firm of chartered accountants were to study the possibility of cash-limiting Family Practitioner Committee budgets (DHSS 1982f). On 19 January 1983 central control of NHS manpower numbers was announced (DHSS 1983e) and on 4 February came the first public suggestion that the Government was seriously considering restrictions on doctors' rights to prescribe (DHSS 1983f); in November 1984 the withdrawal occurred from NHS prescription of a range of proprietary drugs which had been previously freely available (DHSS 1984a). On 8 September 1983, health authorities were instructed to engage in competitive tendering for laundry, domestic, and catering services (DHSS 1983g), and on 19 December the Minister for Health announced proposals to place restrictions on the use of deputising services by off-duty GPs (DHSS 1983h).

THE GRIFFITHS REPORT

On 3 February 1983, towards the conclusion of the spate of initiatives outlined above, a development occurred which was to crystallise and symbolise the post-1982 policy for managing the NHS. The Secretary of State announced that

> Four leading businessmen are to conduct an independent management Inquiry into the effective use and management of manpower and related resources in the National Health Service.... we are setting the Inquiry two main tasks: to examine the way in which resources are used and controlled inside the health service, so as to secure the best value for money and the best possible services for the patient [and] to identify what further management issues need pursuing for these important purposes.... Mr Griffiths has not been asked to prepare a report.... we could simply have set up another Royal Commission and then sat back for several years to await its lengthy report, but on past experience that would not lead to effective action. Instead, we have gone straight for management action, with the minimum of fuss or formality (DHSS 1983i).

Mr Roy Griffiths was Deputy Chairman and Managing Director of Messrs J Sainsbury, and his colleagues the Personnel Director of British Telecommunications (Michael Bett), Group Finance Director of United Biscuits (Jim Blyth) and Chairman of Television South West (Sir Brian Bailey, a former NALGO official).

The Inquiry Team, who conducted their investigation by field visits and discussions rather than by formal hearings, were committed to advise the Government on progress by June 1983, and an interview given to the Health and Social Service Journal during the following month indicated the lines along which they were thinking: concern with the identification of executive responsibility, budgetary reponsibility, and market research of patients' opinions (Halpern 1983). The Team's final report, in the form of a twenty-four page letter (NHS Management Inquiry 1983), was sent to the Secretary of State on 6 October 1983, the full text being made public on 25 October.

The Team's recommendations were baldly stated in eight pages. Firstly, changes within DHSS were proposed: the creation of a Health Services Supervisory Board (chaired by the Secretary of State, and including the Minister for Health, the Permanent Secretary, the Chief Medical Officer, the Chairman [sic] of the NHS Management Board [see below], and two or three non-executive members with general management skills and experience) with strategic reponsibility for the objectives and resources of the NHS, and, responsible to it, a full-time, multiprofessional NHS Management Board to oversee implementation of the strategy (NHS Management Inquiry, 1983 p.3). Hence the Management Board would assume all pre-existing NHS management responsibilities located in DHSS, and its members would include some from outside the Civil and Health Services (p.4). Incentives and sanctions in management were held to require attention, and accordingly great stress was placed on the role of a personnel director as a Board member (pp. 4,7).

Secondly, general managers were proposed for RHA, DHA and Unit levels of organisation; regardless of discipline, such persons were to carry overall management responsibility for achieving the relevant health authority's objectives, and were to have substantial freedom to design local organisational structures. Functionally-based management structures were to be minimised and day-to-day decisions taken at Unit level rather than higher up the organisation (pp. 4-5). Thirdly, the review process (see above) was to be extended to unit level, and efficiency savings (see above) replaced by 'cost-improvement programmes', aimed at reducing costs without impairing services (pp. 4-5).

Fourthly, clinical doctors were to become more involved in local management. The prime vehicle for this was a proposed system of 'management budgets': the allocation of workload-related budgets to consultants (pp. 6-7). The locus of consultant contracts was, however, to remain unchanged (p. 19). Finally, the Report urged that more attention be paid to patients' and community opinion, expressed through both Community Health Councils and market research methods (p. 9). The Report also spoke approvingly of some of the earlier initiatives such as performance indicators, the disposal of surplus property, Rayner Scrutinies, and annual reviews (pp. 1,8,13).

On the same day as the release of the Report, the Secretary of State for Social Services told the House of Commons that the Government welcomed the thrust of the recommendations and accepted those applicable within the DHSS; the remainder were to be the subject of a short period of consultation (DHSS 1983j). In the event, this period included an investigation by the House of Commons Social Services Committee, whose conclusions were by no means wholly supportive (Social Services Committee 1984). In general, the comments of nursing and ancillary staff representative organisations were unfavourable (see Harrison 1988b) whilst those of administrators' and treasurers' organisations were favourable: the views of medical organisations are discussed in Chapter 7 below. Unsurprisingly, most comment was directed at the proposal to appoint general managers.

On 4 June 1984, the Secretary of State promulgated the Government's decisions on the Griffiths Report (DHSS 1984b). Some changes, including those within DHSS and pilot schemes for management budgets, were confirmed as in progress already (p.1), and the principle of individual general managers in place of consensus teams accepted:

....The Management Inquiry Team recommended that the general management function should be clearly vested in one person (at each level) who would take personal responsibility for securing action. We accept this view; and believe that the establishment of a personal and visible responsibility.... is essential to obtain a guaranteed commitment.... for improvement in services.... In reaching this conclusion, we do not undervalue the importance of consensus in a multi-professional organisation like the NHS. But we share the Report's view that consensus, as a management style, will not alone secure effective and timely management action, nor does it necessarily initiate the kind of dynamic approach needed in the health service to ensure the best quality of care and value for money for patients (p.2).

General managers were therefore to be appointed at

Regional, District and Unit levels of organisation
by the end of 1985; the posts were to be open to NHS
managers of all disciplines, to doctors, and to
persons from outside the Service. Appointments
were to be on the basis of fixed-term contracts of
three to five years with renewal for further fixed
terms by mutual agreement and, by implication,
dependent upon an assessment of the incumbent's
performance. Any costs incurred by appointments
were to be offset by savings on other management
costs (Appendix C).

THE POST-GRIFFITHS NHS

The Griffiths Report has therefore been a major
influence on the present organisation structure of
the NHS, though some of its recommendations were
modified in the implementation process, and some
subsequent developments have occurred. The present
structure is summarised in Figure 4.1.

The Health Services Supervisory Board and the NHS
Management Board have taken a slightly different
form from that envisaged in the Griffiths Report.
Pressure from the nursing profession led to the
early addition of the DHSS Chief Nursing Officer to
the Supervisory Board (DHSS 1984c), and only one
non-executive outsider, Mr Griffiths himself, was
appointed (Chaplin 1987 p.2). Mr Victor Paige,
formerly Chairman of the Port of London Authority
was appointed as Chairman of the NHS Management
Board in December 1984 (DHSS 1984d), but resigned
in June 1986 in circumstances which suggested, as
some commentators on the original Griffiths
proposals had feared, that there had been
difficulties in reconciling political and managerial
considerations (DHSS 1986a; Barnard and Harrison
1984) on such issues as efficiency savings and the
closure of nurses' homes (Davies 1986a; Petchey 1986
p.101). A revised arrangement resulted, with the
Minister for Health as Chairman of the Management
Board, (by then Sir) Roy Griffiths as Deputy
Chairman (with direct access to the Prime Minister),
and Mr Len Peach (Personnel Director of Messrs IBM
[UK]) as Chief Executive (DHSS 1986b). The
composition of the Management Board has varied
during 1984 to 1987, with roughly one-third of its
members from commercial backgrounds, one quarter
from the NHS, and the remainder from the Civil
Service (Chaplin 1987 p.2; Health Service Journal,

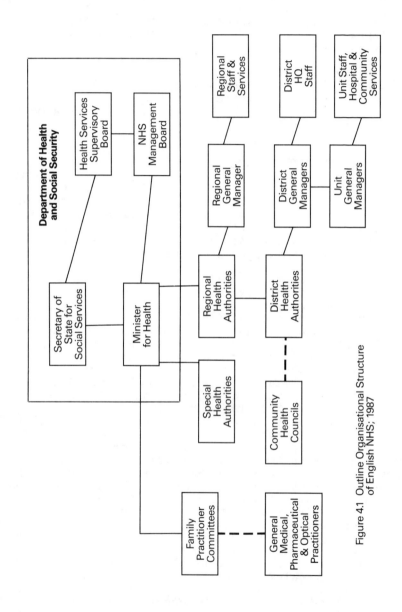

Figure 4.1 Outline Organisational Structure of English NHS; 1987

29 January 1987). The Management and Supervisory Boards remain a part of DHSS rather than separate tiers of management. (For an outline of the internal organisation of DHSS, see Health Trends, 1986, Vol 18, pp. 32-36).

General Managers were appointed by RHAs and DHAs and at Units, though not without suggestions of political 'interference' in ensuring that a number of persons from outside the NHS obtained posts (see, for instance, Timmins 1985). Table 4.1 shows the backgrounds of those appointed up to October 1986. From this it can be seen that more than 60% of posts went to former administrators and treasurers. Many of the doctors appointed were clinicians who undertook a part-time management role at unit level (Sherman 1985 p.152), whilst a significant number of appointments from outside the NHS were retiring officers of the armed forces (see, for instance, Health and Social Service Journal, 12 September 1985). More recent general manager appointments have been on rolling, rather than fixed-term contracts, and a system of individual performance review and performance-related pay introduced (DHSS 1986c; 1986d). The Review Process operates at all levels of the service, and has been modified to consist at regional level of a management meeting between the NHS Management Board and Officers of each RHA at which progress on plans and cost-improvement programmes is reviewed; this is followed by a ministerial meeting with chairpersons of individual RHAs at which more strategic and long-term issues are discussed, along with major issues arising from the management meeting (Mills 1987).

Management budgets have not yet been introduced on a widespread basis. Four health districts were chosen as 'demonstration sites' even before the publication of the Griffiths Report, but despite the involvement of management consultants not all of these were successful at the technical level of establishing the necessary information systems. Moreover, they did not gain the widespread support of clinicians (see, for instance, Arthur Young 1986a; 1986b). A second generation of demonstrations began in 1985; it was intended that this would pay more attention to the behavioural aspects of such systems (DHSS 1985b). Nevertheless, there remained problems in convincing doctors of the value of the innovation and a further set of pilots proved to be necessary; these were launched in November 1986 under the new

Table 4.1   NHS GENERAL MANAGER APPOINTMENTS AND LEAVERS

| FORMER OCCUPATION | APPOINTMENTS AT OCTOBER 1986 | | | | LEAVERS AT MID-1987 |
	REGIONAL GENERAL MANAGER	DISTRICT GENERAL MANAGER	UNIT GENERAL MANAGER	% OF ALL (n=816)	LEAVERS FROM REGIONAL AND DISTRICT LEVELS
NHS ADMIN AND TREASURERS	9	132	364	62%	
DOCTORS (CLINICANS & COMM PHYSICIANS)	1	15	110	15%	2.5% (n = 4)
NURSES	1	4	70	9%	
FROM OUTSIDE NHS	3	38	54	12%	22% (n = 9)
VACANCIES	–	2	13	2%	
TOTAL	14	191	611	100%	

Sources: Syrett (1986)   Peach (1987)

name of 'resource management' (DHSS 1986e). (For a review of the various pilots, see Pollitt et al 1988).

Since 1985, Family Practitioner Committees have been independent of DHAs and RHAs (Allsop and May 1986 p.1). Special Health Authorities now control a number of non-mainstream NHS functions, as well as the London postgraduate teaching hospitals; examples are the NHS Training Authority, the Health Education Authority, and the Prescription Pricing Authority (Alleway and Anderson 1986; Chaplin 1987 p.12 ff). It is by no means clear that organisational changes have now ceased, and at the time of writing consideration is being given to modifications in the area of community care (Millar 1987a).

A final point to be noted, is that the above account of the Griffiths Report reforms relates very much to England rather than to Great Britain as a whole. The general management initiative has been adopted in Wales and Scotland, though with modifications (Scottish Home and Health Department 1985; 1986; Welsh Office 1984a 1984b). Neither performance indicators nor management budgets are as yet used in Scotland.

THE GRIFFITHS DIAGNOSIS

To refer to the Griffiths 'prescription' (above) is to employ a medical analogy which, if sustained, further implies a 'diagnosis'. If Griffiths supplied a prescription for putting the NHS right, then what was wrong? The notion of a diagnosis rolls together two elements which are, at least partly, separable from each other: firstly a set of 'facts', and secondly a value judgement that these are in some way undesirable or unsatisfactory. The scare quotes around the word 'fact' serve to emphasise that facts and values are never wholly separable since the selection of relevant facts is itself the consquence of a value judgement.

In the case of Griffiths, the main elements of the Inquiry Team's diagnosis can be extracted from the second half of the Report itself, which though brief and written in compelling style, sets out some of the reasoning behind the recommendations. Four elements are discernable in this diagnosis.

Firstly, the Team were concerned that individual overall management accountability could not be located:

> ....it appears to us that consensus management can lead to 'lowest common denominator decisions' and to long delays in the management process.... the absolute need to get agreement overshadows the substance of the decision required.... In short, if Florence Nightingale were carrying her lamp through the corridors of the NHS today, she would almost certainly be searching for the people in charge (NHS Management Inquiry 1983, pp. 17, 22).

The character of this analysis as a critique of NHS professionalism is largely veiled by the text itself, though reference is made to the need to ensure that professional functions are 'geared into the overall objectives.... of the general management process' (p.14).

The second aspect of the Team's diagnosis was that 'the machinery of implementation is generally weak' (p.14).

> ....there is no driving force seeking and accepting direct and personal responsibility for developing management plans, securing their implementation and monitoring actual achievement.... certain major initiatives are difficult to implement.... [and] above all.... lack of a general management process means that it is extremely difficult to achieve change.... [A] more thrusting and committed style of management.... is implicit in all our recommendations (pp. 12, 19).

Thirdly, the Inquiry Team drew attention to lack of an orientation towards performance in the Service.

> ....it lacks any real continuous evaluation of its performance.... rarely are precise management objectives set; there is little measurement of health output; clinical evaluation of particular practices is by no means common and ecomomic evaluation of these practices is extremely rare (p.10).

Finally, the Team identified a lack of concern with the views of consumers of health services:

Nor can the NHS display a ready assessment of the effectiveness with which it is meeting the needs and expectations of the people it serves. ....Whether the NHS is meeting the needs of the patient, and the community, and can prove that it is doing so, is open to question (p. 10).

What is striking about these four elements of the Griffiths diagnosis is that, as facts, they correspond very closely to the four propositions derived from the empirical evidence about pre-Griffiths NHS management and set out in Chapter 3 above. This correspondence, along with the relevant items from the Griffiths prescription, is summarised in Table 4.2.

Thus the Griffiths Report sees no one individual in charge of the NHS, whilst the research focusses on the other side of the same coin: the localised power of individual doctors (pluralism). Griffiths identifies what is not happening (plans are often not put into practice) whilst the research observes what is happening (managers are reacting mainly to problems thrust upon them [reactiveness]).

Griffiths notes a failure to set and pursue objectives; the research observes that existing activities are largely taken for granted (incrementalism). Finally, Griffiths points out the lack of managers' attention to patients and the community, whilst the research shows where managers did direct their attention: internally, towards provider groups (introversion). In short, however informal and unstructured their research methods, the Inquiry Team's observations are largely borne out by independent research.

As noted above, however, a diagnosis implies more than just a set of facts. The value judgement entailed by the Griffiths Report is that these facts are undesirable, that the state of affairs which they represent is illegitimate. In other words, for the Inquiry Team, the notion of the NHS manager as diplomat (most recently stated, it will be recalled, in Patients First in late 1979) was by 1983 no longer an acceptable one. The prescription is, of course, aimed at changing this prevailing model of management, and it is possible therefore to infer from it the authors' assumptions about why managerial behaviour had hitherto assumed a

69

Table 4.2   Correspondence of Research Findings and
the Griffiths Analysis

ACADEMIC RESEARCH (see Chap 3)	GRIFFITHS 'DIAGNOSIS'	GRIFFITHS PRESCRIPTION
PLURALISM	LOWEST COMMON DENOMINATOR DECISIONS, NO-ONE IN CHARGE	GENERAL MANAGEMENT IN PLACE OF CONSENSUS
REACTIVENESS	LACK OF CONCERN WITH IMPLEMENTATION	EXTENSION OF REVIEW PROCESS, INCENTIVES FOR MANGERS
INCREMENTALISM	LACK OF PERFORMANCE ORIENTATION	EXTENSION OF REVIEW PROCESS, COST-IMPROVEMENT PROGRAMMES, MANAGEMENT BUDGETS
INTROVERSION	LACK OF ATTENTION TO CONSUMERS	MORE CONCERN WITH CONSUMER, MARKET RESEARCH

diplomatic character; in stressing, as they do, such factors as the need for individual accountability, review, and incentives for managers, they make the managers themselves responsible.

But, as was seen in Chapter 3 above, the research findings about pre-1982 NHS management show that their diplomatic behaviour was related at least as much to their lack of influence over doctors as to the lack of incentive to behave differently. To this extent, therefore, NHS managers have become scapegoats; to invert Stanley Baldwin's well-known attack on the newspaper proprietors ('power without responsibility, the prerogative of the harlot throughout the ages'), responsibility without power characterises the scapegoat (Harrison 1984 p. 17). And indeed it may be added that managerial behaviour outside the NHS may be more pluralistic than the authors of management textbooks would allow (Dalton 1959; Pettigrew 1973; Pfeffer 1978; 1981; Mangham 1979).

CONCLUSION: A CHALLENGE TO THE MEDICAL PROFESSION

But it does not follow from this that the Griffiths prescription and the other contemporary management initiatives discussed above will not have any impact upon doctors. In principle a number of these developments do challenge the medical profession, in two kinds of way. (Doctors' own views of this are discussed in the final Chapter).

Firstly, it is clear that some of the initiatives represent actual or potential challenges to specific aspects of clinical freedom or medical authority, though some (for instance, competitive tendering and the choice of topics for Rayner scrutinies) do not. The clearest examples are perhaps the restrictions on prescribing and the creation of general managers, with the concomitant loss of the profession's veto on management teams. The review process is intended to procure a shift in de facto priorities away from those of the most prestigious sections of the medical profession (the acute specialties) and towards less prestigious areas such as the elderly, mentally ill and mentally handicapped.

Other initiatives provide the opportunity for challenging doctors, if managers choose to take that opportunity. Clinical performance indicators

reflect the way in which hospital consultants manage
their beds and their workload and therefore allows
this limited aspect of their performance to be
visible to others (Shortell et al. 1976). Direct
management access to consumer and community opinion
(through market surveys, for instance) represents a
challenge to the widespread assumption that only
doctors may legitimately speak on behalf of patients
or be aware of their needs. Systems of management
budgets could, if managers choose and if measures of
casemix severity are introduced, be used as a
vehicle for imposing management priorities on
clinicians and for controlling the costs of each
type of case (Harrison 1986 pp. 8-9).

In these ways, the potential for greater managerial
control over doctors has been created: the potential

> to move from a system that is based on the
> mobilisation of consent to one based on the
> management of conflict - from one that has
> conceded the right of groups to veto change to
> one that gives the managers the right to
> override objections (Day and Klein 1983 p.
> 1813).

Thus the Griffiths and related reforms set out to
challenge forty years of professional domination of
the NHS (Petchey 1986 p. 100), though it was not to
be expected that members of the government would put
it in such blunt terms. In opening the House of
Commons debate on the Griffiths Report, the
Secretary of State said

> Of course doctors and nurses will continue to
> make their own decisions about how they treat
> their patients. But equally it would be
> foolish to deny that there are practical
> constraints imposed on consultants in a world
> of necessarily limited resources (House of
> Commons Debates, 4 May 1984, Col. 649).

The truism that clinical freedom cannot be absolute
serves to obscure the fact that it may have degrees.

But as Schulz and Harrison (1983 p. 44) have pointed
out, the potential for influence is not the same as
its employment, and the second way in which
contemporary management reforms threaten the medical
profession is by constraining NHS managers to behave
as agents for the government. Notwithstanding the

ostensible commitment to decentralisation of the
then new government in 1979 (DHSS and Welsh Office
1979), this strategy amounts to one of
centralisation. The main elements of the strategy
are the review process and the associated incentive
system for managers: limited-term contracts
accompanied by performance appraisal and bonus
payments (see above). Further indications of such
centralisation are the emergence in 1985 of an
Inter-Regional Secretariat for Chairmen and General
Managers of RHAs (Alleway 1987a p. 762), and in
1986 of an embryo national management agenda
document from within DHSS (Hyde 1986 p. 374). It
is notable how such strategies have rapidly
overtaken more decentralised attempts to improve
management, such as the management advisory
services promulgated in Patients First (see above,
Chapter 2).

These strategies represent an unprecedented degree
of centralisation in the NHS (Taylor 1984 p. 22),
not just (pace Petchey, 1986 p. 100) a minor twist
in an existing spiral. Indeed, the review process
and incentive arrangements can be seen (especially
in the context of reported ministerial interest in
general manager appointees: Timmins, 1985) as the
creation of a de facto line relationship from NHS
Management Board to Regional General Manager, to
District General Manager to Unit General Manager
(see Figure 4.1) outside the ostensible semi-
independence of health authorities (Klein 1984a, p.
1706).

> At present the NHS is rather like a feudal
> society in which independent authority is
> exercised by a number of groups, notably by the
> medical profession.... The Griffiths proposals
> therefore imply as dramatic a transformation,
> in the direction of a bureaucratically-driven
> national system, as that wrought by the Tudors
> after the Wars of the Roses (Day and Klein
> 1983, p. 1813).

To return to discussion in the terms of Figure 1.2,
NHS managers have become agents of the third party
(government), rather than of the physicians, and the
established influence of the latter is, in principle
at least, under challenge from the enforced new
alliance. Contemporary management reforms in the
NHS represent an attempt to shift the frontier of
control between government and physicians. Such an
analysis bears some resemblance to 'structural

interest theory' (Alford 1975), an approach adopted, though not in any sustained way, in two popular textbooks of British health policy (Ham 1985 pp. 195-197; Allsop 1984 pp. 8-10).

In outline, structural interest theory posits that the field of health care can be conceptualised as consisting of a number of broad interests; whilst each of these may display some internal heterogeneity and even conflict, each is defined in terms of the extent to which its interests are 'served or not served by the way in which they fit into the basic logic and principles by which.... institutions.... operate' (Alford 1975 p. 14). Interests may be 'dominant', 'challenging', or 'repressed'. Dominant interests are those served by the existing order; their strategies are therefore basically defensive, and they may well be buttressed by general societal approval of their status (pp. 14, 17). Challenging interests are created and sustained by macro-level societal changes such as technology and markets; their interests lie in changing the status quo (pp. 14-15). Repressed interests are the opposite of the dominant in that the nature of institutions systematically ensures that they are not served, though from time to time specific pressure groups may arise within the repressed interest, and may achieve isolated changes (pp. 14-15).

In Alford's own case studies of health care in New York City, doctors are seen as a 'professional monopoly', and hence as the dominant interest; the owners and managers of health care institutions, together with relevant government actors and third-party payers, are seen as 'corporate rationalisers', challenging the dominant medical interest with attempts to introduce planning systems and cost controls (pp. 194-209). Finally, the 'community population' is the repressed interest: those members of the public who cannot afford health insurance and yet do not qualify for government welfare benefits (p. 15).

Alford's approach cannot simply be applied to the British NHS without some modification. Fairly obviously, Alford's analysis of the American repressed community population would have to be revised. More importantly, as Chapter 3 has shown (and contrary to what is implied by Ham's and Allsop's references to Alford), it is only very recently that NHS managers have looked likely to challenge doctors, whereas Alford argues that the American corporate rationalisers have been challenging the professional monopoly for some decades. This observation serves to raise the first of the two remaining questions which this book sets out to answer (see Chapter 1 above); why did the British Government begin to mount the challenge to doctors when it did (in about 1982) and in the form represented by the Griffiths and related initiatives? Chapters 5 and 6 address this question, suggesting amongst other things that a somewhat wider range of macro-level factors than those considered by Alford has been at work in shaping the challenge of the British health care corporate rationalisers.

Chapter 5

1982-1984: THE CONTEXT OF HEALTH CARE POLITICS

The purpose of Chapters 5 and 6 is to provide an interpretation of the shift in government policy towards the mangement of doctors and the NHS which has been described in previous Chapters. The interpretation offered is complex, incorporating six major variables whose interaction, it is argued, produced the Griffiths Inquiry and the other managerial innovations outlined in Chapter 4. The present Chapter is concerned to identify and outline these six variables, which are:

. perceptions about Britain's economic performance;
. demographic trends in Britain;
. technological developments;
. public opinion;
. parliamentary actvity; and
. pressure group activity.

These factors are, for the moment, treated in isolation from each other; an attempt to link them into a coherent explanation is made in Chapter 6 below.

This Chapter has a second purpose. It is crucial to the explanation offered in Chapter 6 that the six variables not only existed, but that relevant policymakers (members of the Government and senior civil servants) were aware of them. Hence each of the following sections attempts to demonstrate such awareness. The theoretical implications of this and of other aspects of the explanation offered are discussed in Chapter 6.

BRITAIN'S ECONOMIC PERFORMANCE

Successive Conservative Governments since 1979 have consistently adopted the stance that their first priority was the improvement of Britain's economic performance as a prerequisite for improvements in living standards (see, for instance, Conservative Party 1979, pp. 7-8). In particular, the preconditional status of the national economy for welfare state provision has been consistently stressed by Ministers, including both Secretaries of State for Social Services in the period under examination:

....a sound and thriving economy must be the foundation of all welfare provisions (Mr Patrick Jenkin; DHSS 1979b).

....the Government is determined to stand by its economic policy. This means that health authorities' cash limits will not be increased this year for the effect of excess price inflation.... (Mr Patrick Jenkin, 1979, emphasis original).

....every nation ....must adjust to the economic realities of the time.... the National Health Service is not immune from these realities ... That is why the NHS had to make its contribution to the exercise which the Government undertook [the 'Lawson' cuts'] to bring public expenditure as a whole back to the course which we had planned for it (Mr Norman Fowler; 1983).

Before examining the content of economic policy, it should be noted that perceptions about economic growth are only relevant to health care expenditure if three prior conditions are fulfilled. The first condition is that health care will continue to be mainly publicly financed. In fact despite a general preference for competition and privatisation (Jackson 1985a, p. 26), early suggestions that insurance-based funding might provide an alternative to tax-based finance (see, for instance, DHSS 1981b, p. 2), and surveys of health care financing practices in mainland Europe and the United States (see, for instance, Wintour and Wheen 1982), government spokesmen have, in the period with which this Chapter is concerned, subsequently stressed the continuation of public funding of the NHS:

....the Government have no plans to change the present system of financing the NHS largely from taxation (Mr Norman Fowler, DHSS 1983l).

....[following] detailed consideration of
alternative ways of financing the NHS.... we
are.... committed to the present system....
That statement stands as Government policy
today (Mr Norman Fowler, 1983 pp. 3-4).

A second condition for the relevance of the national
economy to NHS policy is that it must be assumed
that no substantial shifts in government priority
between policy sectors will occur. In other words,
whatever the state of the economy, it is possible in
principle to shift resources from, say, law and
order, into health. Although between 1979 and 1984
the health and personal social services budget grew
at twice the rate of public expenditure as a whole,
most of the differential occurred between 1979/80
and 1980/81. Since then such expenditure has grown
at roughly the same rate as total public expenditure
and slightly more slowly than the main areas of the
welfare state taken together. These trends are
summarised in Table 5.1. No major priority shift
towards the NHS is occurring.

The final condition needed to justify a link between
NHS spending and the economy is for the Government
to be unwilling to raise additional revenue from
increased taxation. And indeed governments since
1979 have consistently stressed their ambition to
reduce the tax burden (Conservative Party 1979
p. 13; 1987 p. 5), and have reduced income tax rates
in part fulfilment of this, though it should be
noted that this may well have been offset by changes
in indirect taxation (Jackson 1985b, p. 57).

These conditions being fulfilled, the question
arises as to what is meant by giving priority to
economic policy over the NHS. An economist of
Keynesian persuasion might, for instance, conclude
that high levels of unemployment should be tackled
by the stimulation of demand through job creation
(Barber 1967 p. 247 ff), perhaps in the public
services. It is clear, however, that this is not a
position which has been adopted by governments in
the last decade. Nairne, a former Permanent
Secretary at the DHSS, notes that from 1975/76 the
then Labour Government had felt it necessary to make
cuts in planned public expenditure in response to
the economic crisis triggered by the 1973-74 energy
crisis (Nairne 1985, p. 121). It is for this reason
that Jackson (1985a p. 29) refers to the Callaghan

1982-1984: THE CONTEXT OF HEALTH CARE POLITICS

TABLE 5.1   Selected Aspects of Public Expenditure: 1979-1984

(Index of expenditure at 1979/80 price levels:
cash figures adjusted by using GDP deflator)

Programme	1979/80	1980/81	1981/82	1982/83	1983/84
Housing	100	83.2	53.1	42.3	46.4
Education and Science	100	102.7	101.5	102.5	103.1
Health & Personal Social Services	100	107.6	109.6	111.6	114.1
Social Security	100	101.8	112.9	120.1	124.9
Sub-Total of above	100	101.2	103.3	106.1	109.4
Total Public Expenditure	100	101.5	104.3	105.9	107.6

Source: Derived from Robinson (1986 p 4)

Government as the first British monetarist administration.

Although there have been deep divisions within the Conservative Party concerning economic strategy (Holmes 1985) the public spending policy of the Governments since 1980 has been largely dominated by attempts to control inflation and boost employment through control of the money supply: the so-called Medium Term Financial Strategy (Henley et al 1986 p. 19). Associated with this strategy has been a concern that government budget deficits would make control of the money supply more difficult; consequently, increasing emphasis has been placed on a fiscal strategy of restricting the Public Sector Borrowing Requirement (PSBR) to a reducing proportion of Gross Domestic Product (GDP) (Jackson 1985b, pp. 51-55). Table 5.2 summarises relevant trends.

It is evident from the Table that the Government experienced difficulty in making forecasts (hence the difference between columns 2 and 3); this was largely due to inaccurate forecasting of unemployment, and hence of benefits payments (Jackson 1985b, p. 53). Hence the progress planned in the 1980 budget was not made (cf columns 2 and 6). The greatest difficulty was experienced, as it transpired, over the period 1980 to 1981, when (see column 5) the absolute GDP was falling. In spite of all this, fiscal policy was extremely tight and the objective of reducing PSBR as a percentage of GDP was eventually met (column 6), even though the original targets were not. Given that the 1981-82 improved figures (columns 5 and 6) would not have been evident before quite late in 1982, the situation in late 1981 and early 1982 would have looked unpromising to policymakers (Thain 1985 p. 275).

It should be reiterated that it is such perceptions of the economic situation on the part of government and senior civil servants that are crucial to the present analysis. The Medium Term Financial Strategy and associated fiscal measures formed part of those perceptions, and the data in Table 5.2 allow a plausible inference to be made about perceptions of the success of the strategy. It is of course the case that the appropriateness of such perceptions have been challenged on various grounds. Thus, on technical grounds, it has been objected that crude PSBR data (that is, not controlled for unemployment levels) are inadequate for the analysis

TABLE 5.2   THE MEDIUM-TERM FINANCIAL STRATEGY

1	2	3	4	5	6
Financial Year	1980 Budget: Target PSBR as % of GDP	Target PSBR as % of GDP (as set at budget preceding Col. 1 date)	PSBR Outturn (£000 million)	GDP Index (1980 = 100)	Outturn PSBR as % of GDP
1979/80	4.75	4.75	9.9	102	5.0
1980/81	3.75	3.75	13.2	100	5.5
1981/82	3.0	4.5	8.6	99	3.5
1982/83	2.75	3.5	8.7	100	3.25

Sources: Columns 2, 3 and 6   Jackson 1985b p.53
           Column 4   Buckland 1987 p.243
           Column 5   Central Statistical Office 1986 p. 94

(Jackson 1985b p. 54), or that the expression of GDP net of privatisation proceeds is misleading (Buckland 1987 p. 242). On ideological grounds, Gough (1979 p. 80) has drawn attention to the value-laden nature of the way in which the economic variables are defined. And a considerable number of commentators have challenged whether any 'crisis' of welfare state expenditure can really be regarded as occurring (Glennerster 1985 p. 248; Davies and Piachaud 1985 p. 95; Gillion and Hemming 1985 p. 35; Hill and Bramley 1986 pp. 87-88). Valid as they may be in themselves, however, such objections are not relevant as explanations of government policy.

DEMOGRAPHIC TRENDS

The population of Great Britain, though it has grown in total continuously since the early Nineteenth Century, is currently growing much more slowly than before; it is expected to increase by only about four percent in the last two decades of the present Century (Central Statistical Office 1983). This is largely the result of two other Twentieth Century trends. Firstly, life expectancy at birth has improved from under fifty years to over seventy for men and almost eighty for women (DHSS 1987 p. 14); secondly, the crude birth rate has tended to fall, albeit with some fluctuations (Central Statistical Office 1983).

The net result of these trends is a population which contains increasing numbers, and proportion, of the elderly. Thus whilst only four percent of the 1901, and eleven percent of the 1951 population were aged sixty-five years or over, the figure for 1981 until the end of the Century is fourteen percent (Central Statistical Office 1983). Within this is another trend which is of particular significance for health policy; the very elderly, that is, of seventy-five years and over, continue to increase in numbers, reaching a plateau of about 3.5 million by 1991 (Central Statistical Office 1983). The particular significance for health policy of this group is that they are disproportionately heavy users of health care resources. Table 5.3 demonstrates the extent of this. The average per capita cost of hospital and community health care for the seventy-five years and over group is almost five times that of the national average (that is, for all ages) or nine times that of persons of working age

TABLE 5.3

Estimated Average Hospital and Community Health Current Expenditure per Head
of Population in 1980-81 and by Age Group (England)

	Total Population	Births	0-4	5-15	16-64	65-74	75 and over
Expenditure per head	£160	£855	£155	£65	£85	£310	£765

Source: DHSS 1983m; reproduced by permission of the Controller of Her
        Majesty's Stationery Office

(DHSS 1983m, pp. 11-12).

The financial consequence for the NHS of this trend is that (all other things equal), annual real growth in resources is required if existing levels of service are to be provided to the increased elderly population. The magnitude of this required real growth varies year by year (DHSS 1983m p. 11; Maynard and Bosanquet 1986 pp. 7-8), but approximates to one percent of the total revenue budget for hospital and community health services. Whilst there has been some dispute about the extent to which such additional demands might be offset by 'efficiency savings' or 'cost-improvement programmes' (see above, Chapter 4, and Travis 1986 p. 1219), it is clear that their existence has long been recognised by policymakers in public speeches and official documents:

.....the rising numbers of the very old in our community daily present us with new problems on a scale that we have only begun dimly to comprehend (Mr Patrick Jenkin; DHSS 1979b).

.....the demand for health care is in effect unlimited, and that is very much accentuated by demographic factors.... (Sir Patrick Nairne, Permanent Secretary, DHSS; Committee of Public Accounts 1981 p. 10).

.....these population changes led to extra need for hospital and community health services.... if the NHS.... had failed to deliver extra services of at least that amount.... standards would have dropped (DHSS 1983m, p. 11).

.....you know better than I do about the increasing pressures arising from demographic factors.... (Sir Kenneth Stowe, Permanent Secretary, DHSS; Stowe 1986 p. 741).

In 1986, the Minister for Health formally recognised the need for one percent per annum growth to meet demographic changes (Social Services Committee 1986 p. xiii).

TECHNOLOGY

The main topic of this section is developing medical 'technology', a term used to signify not just

machinery or equipment, but techniques of diagnosis
and therapy too (Stocking 1985 p. 5); however, a
concluding paragraph discusses the development of
information technology.

Two features of modern medical technology are
important for the present analysis. The first is
that its spread seems to be somewhat difficult to
control. One reason for this is that it generates
quite high expectations on the part of the public
(Stocking 1985 p. 48), and another, possibly
related, is that governments have found it convenient to present developments in such technology
as political achievements (see, for instance, DHSS
1979 c, p. 1; DHSS 1983m, pp. 16-17). Perhaps most
important, however, is that the nature of much of
this technology is such that its initial adoption by
doctors can be concealed from NHS managers;

....innovations.... may have diffused readily
because there was no need to define explicitly
the uses to which staff and equipment were
being put. For example, neural tube defect
screening [that is, for spina bifida] with its
various components of blood tests,
amniocentesis, counselling, and abortion is
costly. However, it seems to have been able to
diffuse relatively rapidly because in its
initial stages in any particular locality, no
new equipment or funds needed to be requested.
It is only as the service builds up that
it becomes necessary to ask for additional
laboratory equipment, etc (Stocking 1985, pp.
67-68).

Indeed the working party responsible for producing
the booklet Expensive Medical Techniques was able to
go so far as to develop a typology of strategies by
which such technological 'cuckoos' turned up in the
health authority 'nest' (Council for Science and
Society 1982, pp. 18-21).

The second important feature about developing
medical technology is that, in general, it is
expensive in itself and is not labour-saving.
Whilst it is not practicable to calculate detailed
costs, Maynard and Bosanquet (1986 p. 8) have
concurred with DHSS estimates that changes in
diagnostic and treatment practices in the acute
sector alone require half of one percent per annum
real increase in the hospital and community health

service budget. As with the demographic changes outlined above, the financial effects of techno-logical change are well known to policymakers (DHSS 1979b p. 1; DHSS 1983m p. 17; Committee of Public Accounts 1981 p. 10), and the figure of half of one percent as the annual real increase in budget necessary to keep pace with such developments was formally recognised by the Minister for Health in 1986 (Social Services Committee 1986 p. xiii).

Information technology has, during the 1980s, become cheaper, more accessible and more familiar to managers and policy makers in the public services as well as in the private sector. One well-known large-scale DHSS application is the computerisation of social security calculations (O'Higgins 1984). Such technology has performed an enabling role in respect of some of the NHS managerial developments outlined in Chapter 4 above. It is hard to imagine, for instance, a system of dispersed management budgets without computerised information (Arthur Young 1986a p. 1), whilst the second, computerised, package of performance indicators was much more 'user-friendly' (and hence, likely to be used) than the original manual of typescript tables (Fairey 1985). The role of such technology in public sector management has been neatly summarised by Pollitt:

> Finally, computers: they have played a significant permissive role in the introduction of performance assessment systems. The advent of dispersed, multi-access systems with cheap desk-top VDUs has permitted the storage, rapid retrieval and display of the vast quantities of data that most performance assessment schemes appear to need. Computers obviously didn't produce the wave [of such schemes in the public sector] but they have allowed it to flow more swiftly and to deposit less paper (Pollitt 1986 p. 160).

PUBLIC OPINION

In considering the impact of public opinion upon government behaviour towards the NHS, it is convenient to separate opinions about the NHS in general from those about specific actors: doctors, bureaucrats, and trade unionists. The evidence cited in this section is derived entirely from opinion polls (and is therefore subject to all the criticisms of polling as a technique: see Taylor-Gooby 1985a p. 74 ff), but does not attempt to give a complete review of relevant findings. Moreover, it has not been possible to show that ministers were aware of these specific findings, though they were certainly aware of the general trends indicated. (The Conservative Party conducts private polls, but the results of these remain confidential for some fifteen years after collection of the data.) For these reasons, this evidence is strongly suggestive rather than wholly conclusive.

Very general poll questions about the popularity or importance of the NHS tend to produce evidence of massive public support; for instance, Taylor-Gooby (1985b p. 76) cites a 1984 poll in which 93 percent of respondents considered the continuation of the Service to be 'very important'. Such general evidence can be objected to, on the grounds both that it takes no account of public opinion about taxation, and that it merely taps attitudes concerning the broad notion of a health service, rather than respondents' concrete experiences with the NHS.

Nevertheless, poll questions concerning NHS finances have also produced responses strongly in favour of additional financial resources for the Service. The British Election Surveys for 1974 and 1979 show, respectively, 84 percent and 87 percent of respondents saying it to be 'very important' or 'fairly important' that more money be provided to the NHS (Sarlvik and Crewe 1983). Similarly, MORI polls throughout the two decades up to 1980 show increasing proportions of respondents (70 percent by 1980) considering 'too little' to be spent on the NHS (New Society, 4 December 1980, pp. 464-465), a finding confirmed in Gallup Polls (Webb and Wybrow 1981 p. 50). The trend continued after 1980 (Economist, 8 October 1983, pp. 18-21), and more recent Marplan polls confirm the implication that extra funds should be derived from additional taxation or from adjustments in government priorities rather than from increased charges (Davies 1987 p. 382). Finally, Taylor-Gooby's 1981 survey of the Medway area seems to confirm the universalistic principle of the NHS, with 66% of respondents saying that services should not be restricted on grounds of income (Taylor-Gooby 1985b pp. 30-31).

Predictably, poll questions which focus on the

Table 5.4   Public Opinion and Health Professionals

February 1980: How would you rate the honesty and
ethical standards of the people in these different
jobs?   Would you say they are high, average or low?
(percentages)

	High	Average	Low	Don't Know
Doctors	73	21	3	3
Members of Parliament	17	49	25	10
Police Officers	51	38	7	4
Trade Union Leaders	10	33	46	11
Business Executives	17	49	19	15
Local Councillors	16	50	24	10
Solicitors	49	33	7	11

Source   MORI/Sunday Times

December 1983: For each [of the following types of
people] would you tell me whether you generally
trust them to tell the truth or not? (percentages)

	Tell Truth	Do Not	Don't Know
Business Leaders	25	65	10
Clergymen/priests	85	11	4
Civil Servants	25	63	12
Doctors	82	14	4
Government Ministers	16	74	10
Journalists	19	73	8
Judges	77	18	5
Ordinary man/woman in the street	57	27	16
Politicians generally	18	75	7
Police	61	32	8
Teachers	79	14	7
Television newsreaders	63	25	11
Trade Union Officials	18	71	11

Source   MORI/Sunday Times

Table 5.4   Public Opinion and Health Professionals
             (cont'd)

May 1987: Which two or three of the groups of people
on this list do you yourself have most respect for?
(percentages)

Civil Servants	3
Company Directors	3
Doctors	70
Journalists	1
Members of Parliament	4
Nurses	75
Policemen	50
Scientists	12
Social Workers	14
Teachers	20
Trade Union Leaders	3
None of these	1
Don't know	2

Notes: All respondents are adults aged 18 and above.
Due to rounding some lines in the 1980 and 1983
Tables do not add to 100 percent. The 1987 Table
contains multiple responses.

Reproduced by permission of Market & Opinion
Research International.

public's actual experiences of the NHS do show some dissatisfactions and specific complaints. Nevertheless, a survey conducted on behalf of the Royal Commission on the National Health Service showed that over 80 percent of inpatients thought the service 'good' or 'very good' (Royal Commission 1979 p. 13), findings subsequently confirmed in a series of polls conducted on behalf of the National Association of Health Authorities (Halpern 1985; 1986; Davies 1987).

In comparison with other occupations, health professionals (doctors and nurses) are held in high public esteem; Table 5.4 summarises the findings of three relevant MORI polls. In the earliest (1980), doctors are easily the most highly rated (in terms of ethics) of a list of occupations, whilst in the second (1987) they are only narrowly beaten as a result of the addition of clerygmen to the list of occupations. In the third (1987), it is the addition of nurses which once more leaves the medical profession narrowly in second place. Since these polls do not ask identical questions or provide identical lists of occupations (no such comparable data are available), they cannot be interpreted as a trend, but they do serve to illustrate the high level of public popularity enjoyed by doctors and nurses. Despite this high level of relative popularity, however, there are some suggestions that public confidence in the medical profession has weakened slightly since the 1960s as a result of greater public exposures to the reports of 'scandals' (Pollitt 1984a), or simply as part of more critical public attitudes towards authority (Harrison et al 1984b).

Public attitudes towards the NHS and to health professionals are, however, unlikely to extend to health service managers and administrators, at least if attitudes to public sector bureaucrats in general are any guide. Thus a MORI poll amongst Southwark residents revealed that 69 percent of respondents felt that the local authority 'wasted' a lot of money, 42 percent that it spent money on the 'wrong things', whilst 7 percent objected more generally to 'bureaucracy' (New Society, 4 December 1980, p. 465). According to the same source, Conservative Party private polls in 1979 revealed similar attitudes nationally.

The same attitude can, of course, be discerned amongst politicians. The constant concern of the House of Commons Select Committees with administrative manpower in the NHS (see below, and, for instance, Committee of Public Accounts 1981 pp. 6-7) is one manifestation of this, whilst others may be found in ministerial speeches:

....if we can slim the management structure of the service, we can switch tens of millions of pounds out of administration and directly into the care and cure of patients (Mr Patrick Jenkin: DHSS 1979d).

Mr Fowler, too, was noted for his slighting references to the NHS's 'administrative tail' (Halpern 1987), a view which is all of a piece with what Fry (1984 p. 325) somewhat euphemistically terms Mrs Thatcher's 'irreverent' attitude towards public servants. Such anti-statism is, however, not a wholly distinctive Conservative view, for politicians of the left (such as Barbara Castle, Richard Crossman and Tony Benn) have also often felt their efforts to have been thwarted by the bureaucracy (Hennessy 1987).

If bureaucrats are unpopular, so were trade unions, at least over the period with which this study is concerned. The public distrust of union officials is evident in Table 5.4 above, whilst other polls show dislike both of unions as organisations and of their activities. Thus, between 1979 and 1980 the proportion of respondents who felt that unions were 'a bad thing' rose from 29 percent to 43 percent (Webb and Wybrow 1981 p. 65), whilst contemporary Gallup polls showed increasing public hostility towards what was perceived as trade union 'political' activity (pp. 67-71). In a 1980 poll, 78 percent of respondents considered that British trade unions had 'too much power' and showed 'too little responsibility' (Times, 21 January 1980). Such data, of course, refer to trade unions in general, but there seems no reason to conclude that they do not apply equally to those unions organising within the NHS.

THE ROLE OF PARLIAMENT

In the early 1980s, the House of Commons became especially interested in the management of the NHS, and particularly in the number of persons employed in it. Some of this interest was from individual Members, one of whom, Mr Ralph Howell, has asked 'hundreds of parliamentary questions.... aimed at proving there is no proper management' in the NHS and recommending that health authorities should have 'Chairmen [sic] with full executive powers' (personal communication 1987; see also Howell 1982). Moreover, at least one of the specific proposed reforms outlined in Chapter 4 reached the political agenda as a result of Members' complaints on behalf of constituents: restriction of GPs' usage of deputising services (DHSS 1983n p. 1). However, it has been House of Commons Select Committees which have been most prominent in castigating the management of the NHS: the Social Services Committee and the Public Accounts Committee.

Select Committees of the House of Commons had existed in various forms since the nineteenth century and had, for much of the twentieth century, been the subject of campaigns for parliamentary reform, being seen as a means of countering an Executive growing in power as a result both of the party system and of the growing technicality and complexity of government concerns. Specialist committees of backbenchers were thus seen as a remedy, and much of the support for such reform was across party lines (Baines 1985 pp. 13-15). Some initial reforms took place under the Labour Goverments of 1964 to 1970, when a mixture of departmental and suject-based committees was established, though these were not widely regarded as successful (p. 22) and were partly replaced in 1971 by an Expenditure Committee divided into functional sub-committees, one of which covered Social Services and Employment.

A subsequent review of this arrangement nevertheless saw it as being insufficiently structured and focussed, and recommended instead a new system involving a committee for each government department (Baines 1985 pp. 27-28). This was accepted in general terms by the then Labour government, but the outcome of the 1979 General Election left it to the incoming Conservative Government to introduce twelve new committees (p. 30). One of these was the Social Services Committee, which had begun operations by January 1980 (p. 32).

The new committees possess the powers of the House

itself, and may therefore send for persons, papers and records, and appoint specialist advisers (Baines 1985 p. 31). Most hearings are in public (Drewry 1985 p. 386), and the committees strive to produce unanimous reports (p. 361). Drewry (1985 p. 392) has concluded that although in general it is hard to isolate the impact of the new committees, they have certainly resulted in the passage of more information both to MPs and to the public and to pressure groups. Giddings (1985 p. 373) has, in addition, pointed out that the mere fact of having to give evidence concentrates the minds of ministers and senior civil servants and can lead to re-appraisal of policies.

The new Social Services Committee in 1980 had DHSS and its associated public bodies (that is, including health authorities) as its terms of reference; Rush 1985 p. 239). In each parliamentary session, the Committee has conducted one major enquiry (the majority having been related to health services), several shorter enquiries, and (unlike several of the other committees) an examination of health and social service expenditure (Rush 1985 p. 239; Robinson 1985 p. 313). Its output from 1980 to 1987 exceeded that of any other select committee (Warden 1987 p. 1299).

In its Third Report for the Session 1979-1980 the Committee made its first examination of DHSS expenditure plans. As part of a general critique of what it saw as a failure by the Department to maintain strategic control of the NHS (Nairne 1983 pp. 250-252), the Report endorsed the need and scope for greater efficiency in the NHS, but went on to comment on the Secretary of State's claims that the expenditure cuts of the preceding year had been partly offset by increasing efficiency:

> We must, however, express forcibly our disquiet that the Department, whilst embracing the rhetoric of greater efficiency, does not appear to be in a position to measure its actual achievement.... we accordingly recommend that the DHSS should give high priority to developing a comprehensive information system which would permit this Committee and the public to assess the effects of changes in expenditure levels or patterns on the quality and scope of services provided (Social Services Committee 1980 p. x).

The Government's reply to the Committee (DHSS 1980c) forcibly rejected the general critique but ostensibly accepted the need for greater monitoring; proposals for doing this, that is stressing decentralised responsibility to the NHS and the creation of Management Advisory Services (see above, Chapter 2), seemed, however, to miss the point that the Committee had made.

The Social Services Committee returned to the attack in the following year; whilst accepting the notion of Management Advisory Services, it drew attention to the dangers of assuming that falling costs per acute case implied increasing efficiency, and went on:

> if the health authorities do not succeed in squeezing out waste, then they may economise by cutting either the scale or quality of the services.... we.... recommend that as a matter of urgency, every effort should be made to find a way to measure the savings flowing from improved efficiency (Social Services Committee 1981 p. xiii).

Again, in 1982, the Committee remarked that 'there is some suspicion that "efficiency savings" are becoming a regular euphemism for "expenditure cuts"' (Social Services Committee 1982 p. xiii), and still in 1986 it remained sceptical:

> Whilst endorsing the Government's determination to improve efficiency and management in the NHS, we recommend that the Government monitor closely the effect on health services of cost-improvement programmes, to ensure that such programmes do not lead to a reduction in overall health care (Social Services Committee 1986 p. xix).

The Social Services Committee had not been alone in showing interest in the management of the National Health Service. In his annual report on the appropriation accounts for 1979-80 the Comptroller and Auditor-General (the statutory auditor of public expenditure, who had for some years progressively developed an interest in value for money audit as opposed to narrow financial propriety: Henley et al 1986 p. 235) noted wide discrepancies in staffing levels and other variables as between health authorities, commenting that his observations raised

.... the question of the right balance, in the interests of economy and efficiency, between the necessary central direction and oversight of the NHS and a system of delegation and discretion appropriate to a locally-based and managed service (quoted in Committee of Public Accounts 1981 p. 1).

The Committee of Public Accounts (PAC), to whom the Comptroller's reports are rendered (Henley et al 1986 p. 251), took up this matter in a series of hearings in the spring of 1981. Throughout these, members of the Committee stressed the NHS's accountability to Parliament and emphasised their perceptions of a lack of DHSS control over health authorities. As one member (Mr Michael Morris) put it to the DHSS Permanent Secretary, Sir Patrick Nairne:

.... you have made it clear to the Committee that Ministers settle the national policies, but it does seem to me.... that the Department has got a very relaxed approach to monitoring the implementation of these policies.... [Y]ou are relying, it seems to me, almost entirely on cash limits as the control from the centre. I am still not clear why it is that the Department is against issuing firm instructions (Committee of Public Accounts 1981 p. 56).

In response, the DHSS witnesses maintained that detailed central control was not necessary, though they referred on several occasions (Committee of Public Accounts 1981 pp. 5, 53-54, 58) to the Korner working group (see above, Chapter 2), implying that this would in due course provide comparative performance data. (The Korner Group's terms of reference make no reference whatever to the development of information for central monitoring purposes: Steering Group on Health Services Information 1982 p. 1).

However, the Committee were apparently finally persuaded of the undesirability of detailed DHSS control, and contented themselves, with a call for greater upward flow of information as a means of monitoring the comparative performance of different health authorities. Their Report concluded that the mere existence of cash limits was not, as DHSS witnesses had argued, sufficient discipline upon health authorities:

....arrangements will be satisfactory in practice only if accountability upwards is matched by a flow of information about the activities of the districts, which will enable the regions, and in turn DHSS, to monitor performance effectively and to take necessary action to remedy any serious deficiencies, or inefficiency, which may develop (Committee of Public Accounts 1981 p. xvii).

By the time the PAC came to review matters again, in the Spring of 1982, the Review Process, Performance Indicator, surplus land, and private audit initiatives had already been announced (see above, Chapter 4). In his announcement of them, the Secretary of State acknowledged that the first two were a response to the Committee's criticisms (DHSS 1982a p. 3). Welcoming the developments, the PAC concluded that much remained to be done and that it would continue to observe progress (Committee of Public Accounts 1982 pp. vii-viii).

In 1984, the Comptroller and Auditor-General's role had been strengthened by making him an officer of the House of Commons, and putting his former Exchequer and Audit Department on a statutory footing (under the National Audit Act, 1983) with the new title of National Audit Office (NAO) (Garrett 1986). Both the PAC and the NAO continued to monitor the NHS closely; in its sixteenth Report for the session 1983-84 the PAC welcomed the management changes of 1982 (see Chapter 4 above) but continued to criticise NHS manpower levels (Committee of Public Accounts 1984 p. xi).

In 1986, the NAO produced a report questioning whether cost-improvements in the NHS had really been achieved without damage to patient services (NAO 1986 p. 9), a matter which was subsequently taken up by the PAC in its forty-second Report for 1985-86 (Committee of Public Accounts 1986). A good deal of adverse publicity, including the naming by an MP of the District Health Authorities where such cuts had occurred, resulted (Davies 1986b p. 850), and (as noted in Chapter 4) this may have contributed to the resignation of Mr Victor Paige from his post as

Chairman of the NHS Management Board. The Committee
concluded:

> We cannot emphasise strongly enough that both
> the NHS and the Department should keep fully to
> their policy that [Cost-Improvement Programmes]
> should not include savings from cuts in
> services.... And we note that, despite their
> increasingly robust scrutiny of CIPs, DHSS
> could not give an absolute assurance that
> service cuts had not been included (Committee
> of Public Accounts 1986 p. x).

In an interview with a journalist, the Chairman of
the PAC, Mr Robert Sheldon, said 'I don't think that
the DHSS has the control over the NHS that we would
wish to see.... the Department should have greater
control over the hospitals [sic] than it has now.
But I think we are beginning to see improvements'
(Davies 1985 p. 1399). It seems quite clear that
the DHSS's introduction of the Review Process and of
Performance Indicators, and hence its general drift
towards more centralised managerial control over the
NHS, was triggered by the need to respond to House
of Commons criticisms. This is an interpretation
shared by one of the Department's Permanent
Secretaries of the period (Nairne 1985 p. 121),
other senior civil servants, and by District
Administrators in the NHS (Pollitt 1985a p. 3).
Indeed the introduction of these initiatives shows
remarkable opportunism under political pressure.
The Review Process had begun as a local experiment
in one NHS Region, and was seized upon as a more
general answer to PAC criticisms. Similarly, the
decision to create Performance Indicators by
cobbling together extant data from routine statistical returns, was taken within DHSS as a
more-or-less instant response to the problem of how
to compare one health authority with another.

PRESSURE GROUP ACTIVITY

Pressure group activity cannot on its own stand as a
plausible explanation for anything; since such
activity persists continuously in most spheres of
British government, the task becomes one of explaining why some such activity is apparently successful,
whilst some is not. Consequently, a number of
writers such as Solesbury (1976) and Kingdon (1984)
have attempted to identify the determinants of

success in placing particular issues on the political 'agenda'. One variable identified in such writing is timing; sometimes conditions become temporarily favourable for persuading politicans that a particular problem is important (Solesbury 1976 pp. 384 ff; Kingdon 1984 pp. 173 ff). One such policy 'window' (to use Kingdon's terminology) occurs with a change of government, and it is clear that a number of groups saw in the election of a Conservative government in 1979 the opportunity to press their various interests in relation to the NHS.

Thus, the decision in 1982 to experiment with private audit of the NHS (see Chapter 4 above) was a response to pressure from the Institute of Chartered Accountants (DHSS 1982b). Similarly, the then Minister of Health, Dr Gerard Vaughan, was lobbied by the Association of British Launderers and Cleaners and the British Textile Rental Association in the autumn of 1979 (Ascher 1987 p. 26). When it subsequently became evident that NHS managers remained hostile to the Associations' proposals for NHS laundry and linen services to be subcontracted, further lobbying took place in 1981 through the health service press, and involved a wider range of trade associations who stood to benefit from such subcontracting (p. 27). Such industry representatives have continued to argue that they are being unfairly treated even in the system of compulsory competitive tendering outlined in Chapter 4 (Public Service Review, no. 4, 1985 pp. 2,4).

Yet not all pressure groups were concerned with narrow economic interests. Prior to the 1979 General Election, Mr Patrick Jenkin (then Opposition spokesman on Social Services) had conducted informal consultations with a group of NHS Administrators of varying political persuasions. This group had not pressed for the abolition of consensus decisionmaking, but rather for greater delegation and the abolition of the Area tier of organisation.

At a more general level, the Confederation of British Industry (CBI) (the major national employers' organisation) had been criticising government policy on public expenditure. It believed that restrictions beyond those contemplated at the beginning of the Conservative period of office were required in order to provide resources for greater business tax cuts and increased infrastructural capital spending. A systematic statement of this view was set out in a document of 1981 (CBI Working Party 1981) in which it was argued, inter alia, that NHS manpower numbers were excessive and geographically inconsistent (p. 2). It recommended freezing a large proportion of non-direct care posts as they became vacant, the extension of competitive tendering, and the extension of Rayner Scrutinies (pp. 26 ff).

Responding to Parliamentary and industrial concerns about NHS manpower levels, the Secretary of State for Social Services informed the Conservative Party Conference on 6 October 1982 that

....we want manpower directed at serving the patient, not at building new empires of paper and bureaucracy.... I intend to establish a small team, headed by people from private industry, to achieve it. Their job will not be to produce a lengthy report - there is no shortage of lengthy reports in the Health Service - but to help us produce results, not in years, but in months (Fowler 1982 p 12).

Chapter 6

THE POLICY SHIFT: AN INTERPRETATION

A FICTION

The following account is no more than a device for compression and dramatisation of a process of policy emergence that occurred throughout 1981 and 1982. It is (emphatically) not claimed that the following address, or anything like it was ever made by Mr Fowler. It is a <u>logical</u> construction, a way of linking the factors de<u>scribe</u>d discretely in Chapter 5 above, not an empirical account. Nevertheless, it presents a plausible account of the constraints as they might have affected policymakers. The scene is set sometime in late 1982; the Secretary of State for Social Services is addressing junior ministerial colleagues on his proposed strategy for managing the NHS.

Well, colleagues, let me summarise the position in which we find ourselves. The first major consideration is that there are increasing demands being placed upon the NHS; these stem from the increasing number of the elderly in the British population, and the continued development of medical technology. Together, they impose an apparent need to expand the hospital and community health services at somewhere between one percent and one-and-a-half percent per annum in real terms for much of the next decade.

It seems, however, most unlikely that these demands can, or should, be met by a simple expansion of the NHS's budget. Political priorities, such as law and order, and unavoidable commitments, such as the necessity to meet benefit payments for a rising number of unemployed, preclude any wholesale shift of Government priorities and consequent reallocation of existing expenditure in favour of the NHS. We have already investigated the possibility of a change in the funding arrangements for the Service and decided that the present system should be preserved, and our desire to see substantial expansion in the private health care sector has not really been fulfilled. And our Medium Term Financial Strategy means that, far from contemplating an increase in NHS funding, we really should make cuts in accordance with the overall priority which we have given to economic policy.

I am not, of course, going to conclude that such cuts in the NHS should occur. Quite apart from the need to defend the interests of this Department in Cabinet, it seems to me that the Government should recognise the popularity of the NHS with the public. At a minimum, to cut the NHS, which we know to be one of the most popular areas of the welfare state, and a source of satisfaction to most of its users, is to offer the Opposition parties ammunition on a plate at a time when we expect a General Election within twelve months. That is why the Prime Minster has made it clear that the NHS 'is safe in our hands' [Wintour and Wheen 1982 p. 10].

Now none of this prevents us from doing something about the hospital Ancillary workers whose militancy has caused us such problems in the past. Our encouragement of health authorities to introduce competitive tendering for catering, cleaning and laundry has encountered substantial management hostility, according to the industry associations concerned. We shall therefore make it compulsory for authorities to engage in such competition. As a result, I expect that we shall be able to make some financial savings as well as to weaken the hold of the trade unions involved. I also expect that we shall be able to pursue this policy without alienating public opinion, which, in general, has been moving against the unions in recent years; after all, when the public thinks of the NHS, it is doctors and nurses that come to mind, not cleaners and kitchen staff.

But all this is relatively marginal to the central dilemma which I have outlined:

increasing demand for health services in a situation where economic policy demands one course of action, yet political considerations dictate another. The only logical escape from the horns of this dilemma is to make the NHS more efficient: to have our cake and eat it too by keeping tight control of expenditure, but telling the public that it is nevertheless going to get the additional services it demands, through greater value for money.

The ideal strategy for this exists already, through the medium of the 'efficiency savings' which the Government introduced last year. I say that it is ideal because it fully accords with what Professor Klein has described as the strategy of postwar governments: to centralise the credit for what are perceived as successful policies and to diffuse the blame for what is less successful [Klein 1983 p. 140]. The combination of efficiency savings and tight Government control of NHS spending through cash limits means that we can claim the credit for the redistribution of savings made in non-patient areas and diverted back into patient care [see, for instance, DHSS 1985c p. 1]. At the same time, as my predecessor Mr Jenkin made clear [DHSS 1979e], we cannot be expected to tell individual Health Authorities or local managers how to make these savings; they are at the grass roots and are supposed to know best. And they will take the blame for any unpopular changes.

I wish that I could leave it at this. I cannot do so, because of the constant intervention of Select Committees of the House of Commons. Neither the Public Accounts Committee nor the Social Services Committee has been prepared to accept that DHSS control of the NHS is adequate, or that the system of cash limits is sufficient to ensure that NHS manpower only grows in accordance with service needs. Consequently, we have found ourselves pushed down the road of increasingly centralised control of the NHS through devices such as the Review Process and Performance Indicators. Of course, this is made technically easier by the availability of information technology, but it has left us in the position of having to exercise greater control over the NHS than we might have wished.

In spite of this, criticism of NHS staffing levels from both Parliament and the CBI has continued to such an extent that, as you are aware, I have found it necessary to commit myself to the establishment of an inquiry into them. In setting up this inquiry, we have experienced some difficulty in finding someone from industry to take the chair. One senior figure with NHS connections has already declined the position, and we have now approached a Mr Roy Griffiths, Deputy Chairman and Managing Director of Sainsbury's to undertake the role. Although Mr Griffiths has no experience of public services, we are assured that his reputation as an architect of his company's success is a very considerable one. Moreover, the appointment of such a figure ought to satisfy the CBI.

You may be surprised to learn that Mr Griffiths has declined our approach in the terms in which it was made. He is apparently unwilling to chair an inquiry into staffing levels alone. He says that, in his experience, poor control of manpower is a symptom of more general problems in management. Consequently he is only willing to chair a management rather than a manpower inquiry.

I intend to accept Mr Griffiths' suggestion. We clearly, therefore, have to accept the possibility that his inquiry may result in yet further changes in the management structure of the NHS. This would not necessarily be politically damaging, since we should once again be seen to be taking action, and because there is no public sympathy for bureaucrats (any more than there is Government sympathy for them), and it will not matter if some of them are displaced or have to apply for what they regard as their own jobs for the fourth time in ten years. We shall, of course, have to keep a careful eye on the reaction of the medical profession to any changes, though presumably they are not over-fond of bureaucrats either. On the other hand, should Mr Griffiths attempt to strengthen management control over doctors, we can take heart from the fact that their esteem with the public is not as great as it once was.

I hope, colleagues, that you will concur with my analysis.

TESTING THE INTERPRETATION

Can this interpretation be tested in any way? It certainly fits the known facts. But alternative explanations seem superfically plausible too. For instance, Conservative Party ideology is sometimes used to explain what is seen as a generalised attack on the public services (Petchey 1986). Alternatively, all the reforms outlined in Chapter 4 above took place whilst Mr Fowler was Secretary of State for Social Services and Sir Kenneth Stowe was Permanent Secretary at DHSS; might not the change in policy be explained in terms of these individuals' personal views of the situation? These alternative explanations can be investigated by examination of a number of comparisons; whilst even positivist philosophers of science accept that it is in principle impossible to provide conclusive proof of the correctness of any explanation (Popper 1972 p. 172), the proposed interpretation would be strengthened by the elimination of rival interpretations

The timing of the new management initiatives clearly casts serious doubt on any attempt to explain them purely in terms of generalised Conservative ideology or of Mrs Thatcher's reputed orientation towards action rather than reflection, though indeed they are consonant with such ideology. As was noted in Chapter 4 above, policy early in the life of the Conservative Government provided for the continuation of clinical freedom, as espoused by earlier governments. Rather than 1979 (when the Conservatives returned to office), it is the beginning of 1982 which marks the break in policy continuity; from then on, policy towards NHS management becomes interventionist in detail, through such measures as Performance Indicators and the Griffiths changes, in comparison with the earlier less detailed interventions such as cash limits. The events of 1982 onwards contrast sharply with previous ministerial statements such as

> The Government wants to see a simpler, more
> flexible structure in the NHS, with local
> health authorities using their own initiatives
> to respond to local needs, rather than being a
> conveyor for detailed orders and advice from
> the centre (Mr Patrick Jenkin: DHSS 1979f).

Moreover, political parties other than the
Conservatives have not been unfavourable to policies
aimed at more efficient management of the public
services. Robinson and Webb (1987 p. 21) note that
the keenest exponent of the Financial Management
Initiative in central government was a Labour MP,
whilst during General Election campaigns both Labour
and the Alliance parties seemed not to wish to be
seen as opposed to better public sector management
(Davidson 1983; Davies 1986c; SDP/Liberal Alliance
1987 p. 11). It is hardly surprising that the DHSS
Permanent Secretary of the period in question
reminisced as follows:

> I have seen several changes of party in
> government, and changes of administration as
> one Prime Minister from the same party
> succeeded another.... I cannot honestly think
> of any circumstances in which techniques of
> management changed as a result (Stowe 1986 p.
> 739).

Indeed, there is nothing uniquely British about a
perceived need by government to contain health care
expenditure (Gillion and Hemming 1985 pp. 32-33) or
to do so by achieving detailed control over health
institutions' performance through such devices as
diagnosis related groups (Rodrigues 1987).

Nor has Conservative economic policy been distinctive. Despite the popular association of monetarist
economic policies with the 'new right' (Jackson
1985a pp. 26-37), and despite the fact that the
detail of the Medium-Term Financial Strategy was
devised in the Thatcher Government, the general
approach to economic policy which treats monetary
trends as of great importance has been unchanged
since the mid-1970s;

> The Conservative Government of 1979 was not....
> responsible for introducing a monetarist
> counter-revolution in stabilisation policy. It
> continued the policies of its predecessor
> (Gamble and Walkland 1984 p. 80; see also

Keegan and Pennant-Rea 1979 p. 24: Jordan and
Richardson 1987 p. 214 ff).

These observations are consonant with Klein's
comments about party ideology in Britain; 'there is
an inverse relation between the ideological content
of policy and the importance of the policy area
itself' (Klein 1984b pp. 103-104). Party ideology
is not a plausible explanation of the events
outlined in Chapter 4.

A second alternative possible explanation for the
policy shift of 1982 onwards concerns the inclinations of the personalities involved. Both the
Secretary of State (Mr Fowler) and the Permanent
Secretary (Sir Kenneth Stowe) at DHSS came into post
within a short time of each other in the autumn of
1981, following, respectively, the translation of Mr
Jenkin to the Secretaryship of State for Industry,
and the retirement of Sir Patrick Nairne. Might not
one or both of these actors had, for some
bureaucratic-political reason, a more centralist
approach to the NHS?

Whilst it is impossible to be conclusive, the evidence suggests otherwise. Mr Jenkin remained in the
Cabinet throughout his successor's tenure at DHSS
and himself introduced into the Department of
Industry arrangements which included a detailed management information system (Wilks 1985 p. 135). The
two Permanent Secretaries did indeed have rather
different backgrounds, with Sir Kenneth's career,
unlike that of his predecessor, having included
experience in a management services role and in
Departments with a strong executive role. However,
their public statements, at least, seem
indistinguishable in intent from each other's:

> The formulation of Departmental policy plans
> has always been open to misunderstanding as an
> administrative tool, particularly when it has
> suggested a degree of central control that
> cannot be applied (Nairne 1983 p. 250).

> .... if the objectives of health care are to be
> redefined in a constrained environment, they
> must be professionally led, without which we
> get into terrible tangles (Stowe 1986 p. 741).

THE POLICY SHIFT: AN INTERPRETATION

Neither statement is that of an unremitting
centralist. Moreover, work on some of the 1982
initiatives had commenced before Sir Patrick's
retirement. In summary, then, and unlike in Allen's
(1979) study of the Hospital Plan, and Pollitt's
(1984b) study of changes in the structure of
Whitehall Departments, there is a good deal of
evidence which runs against the explanation of
government policy on NHS management in terms of the
personal inclinations of senior actors.

INTERPRETING THE POLICY SHIFT: TOWARDS SOME
CONCLUSIONS

The most obvious alternative explanations for the
change in policy therefore have serious weaknesses,
which have the effect of making the explanation
offered in this Chapter more plausible. However,
this favoured explanation, as has been seen,
involves a number of variables; it is arguably
necessary, therefore, to consider which of these are
necessary conditions, that is that, without them,
the development of Government policy towards the
management of the health service would have been
markedly different. At least five of the factors
appear to fall into this category.

Firstly, it is clear that, without the perception
that the needs of the British economy required
restraint in public expenditure, the managerial
initiatives of 1982 to 1984 would not have occurred.
Thus, such a perception was a necessary condition,
though not a sufficient one, since the intellectual
origins of monetarism reach back over ninety years
(Dunleavy and O'Leary 1987 p. 86), and it has been
shown in Chapter 5 above that it has been the
received wisdom of politicians from both Labour and
Conservative Parties since long before the events
with which this study is concerned. (To ask how
monetarism became the received wisdom would be a
different study, but it may be noted that one
plausible explanation is that given by Kreiger [1986
pp. 190, 296], who argues that post-1973 oil crisis
economic policy in Britain and America developed in
response to a recognition that Keynesian policies
had failed to secure international economic
effectiveness, and hence stable domestic trends.)

Secondly, it also seems clear that, had the NHS not
been a popular area of welfare state expenditure,

financial cuts would have been possible in the same way as in, for instance, housing. There would then have been less necessity to pursue a policy of ostensibly increasing efficiency. In Kreiger's words

> Thatcher has highlighted for destruction programmes that divide the population, leaving the classic universalistic or life-cycle programmes (like the NHS or old-age pensions) more or less intact (Kreiger 1986 p. 96; see also MacGregor 1985 p. 233).

And moreover, health professional workers have not had imposed upon them revised conditions of service in the same way as have professionals in education (cf. Carvel and Perera 1988 p. 30 with Fredman and Morris 1987).

Thirdly, the role of Parliament, especially the Social Services Committee and the Public Accounts Committee, seems to have been a necessary condition in the determination of the form of the efficiency strategy for the NHS. Although there may well have been other factors pushing towards increasing centralisation of control over health authorities (such as Mr Jenkin's difficulties with Lambeth, Southwark and Lewisham Area Health Authority; see DHSS 1980d), it seems that without the constant attention paid by these two committees to the NHS, and without their constant allegations of the lack of Departmental control over manpower, the Government would have been content with cash limits and the continued control of administrative staffing. There would have been no need for performance indicators, the review process, or for any inquiry to be established. It is notable in this context that the most significant Public Accounts Committee critique of lack of central control (Committee of Public Accounts 1981 p. xvii) related only to England, where, unlike in Scotland, performance indicators and the review process were introduced in response.

A non-NHS example of the influence of such committees upon management arrangements is provided by the Treasury and Civil Service Committee which, in 1982, was a major stimulus to the introduction of the Financial Management Initiative in the Civil Service (Gray and Jenkins 1984 p. 418). Such a conclusion about the influence of Select Committees

stands in marked contrast to those of other studies
(see, for instance, Garrett 1986; Drewry 1985).

Fourthly, Mr Griffiths himself was probably a
necessary condition for the recommendations of his
Report. Though his appointment seems to have been
part of an unplanned chain of events, it is likely
that any other chairperson of such an inquiry would
have accepted the original proposed terms of
reference, and confined his or her recommendations
to NHS staffing.

Finally, the availability of information technology
was a necessary condition for those developments,
such as performance indicators and management
budgets, which required the handling and presentation of considerable amounts of data. The lack of
impact of the early, non-computerised, performance
indicators serves as an illustration of this point.

The status of the demographic and medical-
technological variables seems to be secondary. They
certainly served to focus attention on the proba-
bility of increased demand for health care
resources, but it is quite possible that, without
them, the conflict of economic policy and NHS
popularity with the public would still have led to
an 'efficiency' strategy. They are not, therefore,
such obviously necessary conditions as those
discussed above.

To sum up, then, the policy shift away from a
decentralised 'diplomat' model of NHS management
and towards a more centralised and assertive style,
has been interpreted as occurring in a situation
where policymakers were surrounded by constraints
which left little room for a strategy other than the
one which was adopted. They chose ever-increasing
involvement in the detail of health authority
management. Given these constraints, and their
perception by the actors involved, it is difficult
to imagine alternative 'possible worlds' (Elster
1978 pp. 176-176).

SOME THEORETICAL IMPLICATIONS

This study has identified five factors as necessary
conditions for the managerial developments on which
it has focussed. Yet none of these factors was
alone a sufficient condition; rather, the sufficient

condition was the combination of the five. This final section attempts to expand on the theoretical implications of such a mode of explanation.

It will already be clear to the reader that the explanation offered above cannot be neatly accommodated within any one of the three theoretical approaches (ideological corporatism, structural interest theory, and partisan mutual adjustment) discussed in earlier chapters. Indeed, a variable identified in the preceding section as being of considerable importance is one which is normally associated with a different theoretical approach entirely. It is characteristic of the various forms of marxist theory of the state to give explanatory primacy to economic factors in general, and in particular to the need to maintain favourable conditions for the continuation of capitalism.

Such theories generally proceed from the axioms that a capitalist state, in order to survive as such, must perform as least two functions. The first of these is to facilitate 'capital accumulation' and the continuing operation of the capitalist mode of production. This is done by socialising certain forms of expenditure (such as educational infrastructures) which no single capitalist could afford (O'Connor 1973 p. 124 ff). The second essential function posited for the state is the legitimation of the capitalist system in the eyes of its citizens; hence welfare state expenditure in such areas as health care and income maintenance is a way of promoting social harmony (O'Connor 1973 p. 150). Some areas of expenditure might contribute to both functions (Offe 1984 p. 184); the British NHS was intended both to provide a healthy workforce, and to respond to political demands at the end of a major war (Watkin 1978 pp. 2-3). Thus, welfare state expenditure has a natural tendency to rise in line with interest group demands (O'Connor 1973 p. 9) and changing demographic patterns (Wassenberg 1977 p. 80).

Economic decline, however, exposes a tension, or contradiction, between these two functions. Such a decline tends to increase state welfare expenditure and to render the 'legitimation function' increasingly crucial. But at the same time the increase in expenditure threatens capitalist accumulation because capitalists believe (and it is a self-fulfilling prophecy) that growing public expenditure 'crowds out' private investment (Offe 1984 pp. 149-151) and/or encourages inflation (Gough 1979 p. 126). Hence marxists hold that in such circumstances there is a 'crisis of the welfare state'; as Offe puts it, capitalism cannot survive without the welfare state, but cannot survive with it (1984 p. 153).

This final step in the argument is, however, rather weak. Whilst no government can ignore the pressure of international capitalism (since to do so will have adverse economic effects in a capitalist world: Gough 1979 p. 3; Taylor-Gooby and Dale 1981 p. 48), and whilst the loss of citizen perceptions of legitimacy risks public alienation and non-cooperation with the authorities, it does not follow that economic decline will produce the predicted crisis or irreconcilable contradiction. Whilst welfare states almost certainly do help to legitimise capitalism, it does not follow that there is a linear relationship between expenditure in this area and the degree of legitimacy which it provides. In other words, faced with the tension outlined above, governments can pursue strategies aimed at reconciling the situation; as several marxist commentators hve recognised, one cannot assume that an economic situation alone determines events (Gough 1979 p. 32; Miliband 1977 pp. 96-106).

It is then possible to identify a number of alternative strategies which, logically, are available to governments as a means of retaining the legitimacy provided by a welfare state, whilst maintaining expenditure at a level low enough to retain the confidence of capitalists. One such possibility is to seek to convince capitalists that welfare state expenditure is being controlled, so that it need not create any disincentive to invest; to the extent that such a policy convinces capitalists, it will succeed, since, as noted above, their beliefs will be self-fulfilling. It follows, then, that symbolic action on the part of government may be enough: control of politically salient trends such as administrative manpower or the establishment of committees of inquiry.

A second possible government strategy is to increase the (perceived or real) efficiency of the welfare state (Offe 1984 p. 155): to reduce spending whilst maintaining the level of services, or to increase the level of services obtained for existing expendi-

111

ture levels. In effect, this would change the cost/legitimation ratio: to continue to satisfy both capitalists and citizens and to avoid the dilemma otherwise posed by economic decline. Here again, symbolic action may be sufficient, since all that matter are the perceptions of capitalists and citizens. A variant of this strategy would be to reduce the real wage levels of employees of welfare state institutions.

A third available strategy would be to delegitimise some sections of the welfare state, that is, to change public perception to a view that is being 'abused' and is therefore undermining, rather than reinforcing, social harmony. The fact that some sections of the welfare state are known to enjoy rather less popularity than others (Taylor-Gooby 1985a; 1985b) provides a ready opportunity for a government strategy of differential cutting of resources by such means as entitlement reviews, restructuring of benefits, and pursuit of alleged 'scroungers'. In Johnson's words

> the incrementalism that allowed the welfare state to grow so silently is now used to effect its quiet contraction. A touch of privatisation here, a reduction of board and lodging allowance there, a de-indexation of benefit payments, a 'tightening-up' of supplementary benefit qualifications - the multiplicity of these individually small administrative changes amounts to a concerted, yet concealed, contraction of the welfare state (Johnson 1986 p. 461).

Finally, a fourth possible strategy would be to emphasise those parts of the welfare state thought to be important for capital accumulation (such as technical and vocational training) at the expense of those parts not so perceived (such as arts courses). The four strategies are, of course, not mutually exclusive, and all of them can be observed in recent British Government strategy towards the welfare state as a whole.

So long as it is modified so as not to require an irreconcilable crisis of the welfare state, marxist theory can therefore provide a primary account of why the pre-1982 situation of 'ideological corporatism' (Dunleavy 1981) in the NHS has been transformed into one of challenge by the 'corporate

112

rationalisers' (Alford 1975); perceptions of the NHS as a potential obstacle to economic policy, combined with its status as the most popular institution of the welfare state, left available only the strategy of changing the cost/legitimacy ratio by improving the real or apparent efficiency of the Service.

Yet even such a modified marxist approach does not fully account for the events outlined in Chapter 4 above; even within the constraints which the theory posits, policymakers were still left with a choice about the precise nature of, and mechanism for, the efficiency strategy. These choices were, in the the end, largely made for them, pre-empted by the activities of pressure groups and legislators, and finally determined by the accident of Mr Griffiths' chairmanship of the inquiry.

Such micro-level factors are not normally treated as important within marxist theorising, so that, to complete the explanation of the management initia- tives of 1982-83, it is necessary to turn back to a body of theory touched upon in Chapter 3 above. Lindblom (1979 p. 522), it will be recalled, referred to 'partisan mutual adjustment' as a process of interaction where actions of participants affect actions of others, producing outcomes which differ from the intentions of any single actor. Similar notions of reactive, unplanned, and unpre- dictable outcomes are also evident in the 'bounded rationality' theories of H.A. Simon (1957a; 1957b; 1959), subsequently developed into the idea that

> an organisation is a collection of choices looking for problems, issues and feelings looking for decision situations in which they might be aired, solutions looking for issues to which they might be an answer, and decisionmakers looking for work (Cohen et al 1972 p. 2; see also Cyert and March 1963).

Amongst the most recent theorising in this vein is the work of Kingdon (1984) in accounting for how particular issues come to be on government agendas, and how particular policies come to be adopted. Kingdon conceptualises a political system as having three largely, independent, 'streams' flowing through it: problems, policies and politics (p. 20). Problems are dissatisfactions which are brought to the attention of government (p. 95), policy

proposals often exist amongst pressure groups and in
academia long before they are ever linked to any
particular problem (pp. 122-123), whilst the national political picture, in terms of such factors as
dominant ideologies, may be quite unaffected by
either of the other streams (p. 152). Kingdon goes
on to argue, using evidence from the United States,
that it is only when the three streams are 'coupled'
(sic) that substantial likelihood of policy change
occurs (p. 21).

There are some obvious parallels between such a
theoretical approach and the events with which this
book is concerned. Parliamentary and industrial
dissatisfaction about the perceived lack of
government control over health service manpower had
continued for two or three years. Whilst a
Conservative government might be expected to be
ideologically sensitive to such criticism, it was
the 1982 Party Conference that provided the window
of opportunity. The 'policy stream' was of greater
antiquity; as Chapter 2 above has shown, the general
manager/chief executive solution had been canvassed
for many years, though, as Chapter 5 has shown, it
had few advocates in NHS-related circles by 1982.
But this solution was, in effect, revived by Mr
Griffiths' appointment; businessmen are likely to
offer 'businesslike' solutions to problems.

Throughout all the above theoretical discussion, one
theme has recurred, in connection with each theory:
the importance of actors' perceptions of situations.
Thus, it has been noted that macroeconomic trends
are crucially the product of such perceptions (see
also Keegan and Pennant-Rea 1979 pp. 131-137; Ward
1987 pp. 596-597), and that the public popularity of
the NHS can only be a constraint on policy if
policymakers are aware of it. And perceptions of
the legitimacy of the 'medical model' of health and
disease (Ham 1982 pp. 157-159) were crucial in
sustaining 'ideological corporatism'. The role of
perceptions in explanations of policy has been
theorised by Young (1977 p. 3), whose notion of the
'assumptive world' signifies an actor's perceptions
of his or her environment, perceptions which consist
of an intermingling of values, 'facts', and causal
beliefs;

> While the world of immediate experience is
> chaotic.... and ultimately incomprehensible,
> the assumptive world.... imposes order by

simplification, selection, and generalisation. It condenses raw experience into meaning (Young and Mills 1983 p. 17).

Young argues that the elements of an assumptive world are hierarchically ordered; ideology is a general representation of the world and the actor's orientation to it, attitudes are consistencies in the way in which an actor interacts with the world, whilst opinions concern specific day-to-day encounters (1977 p. 7). The results of an actor's interaction with his or her environment are validated by this hierarchy, and dissonance between the interaction and any element of the assumptive world will result either in a change of opinion (attitudes rarely, ideology hardly ever), or in action upon the environment (p. 8). Moreover, the assumptive world also implies a view about how the world ought to be, and hence Young and Mills (1983 pp. 17-18) argue that the link between the material world of ideas is constituted as a reaction to the threat of impending dissatisfaction. 'The nature... of interventive choice can therefore be understood as action to avert the unacceptable' (Young and Mills 1983 p. 126). Research into decisionmaking about public policy is therefore research into the social process by which some set of facts becomes perceived as a problem (1983 p. 20), and Young therefore indicates that specific enquiry into assumptive worlds is necessary; to infer then from behaviour would be tautological. In principle, any data collection methods can be used to do this, but in practice Young favours the conversational inter- view and the use of unobtrusive measures such as speeches or documents written by the actor (1977 p. 3). Finally, assumptive worlds need to be investigated in their context, not in the abstract (1977 p. 16); 'any account of how policymakers make sense of circumstances must also establish what those circumstances are' (Young and Mills 1983 p. 24).

In general, then, the theoretical implications of the present study are summed up in McKay and Cox's remark that

> Social and economic forces.... precipitate the environment in which problems arise and to which.... ideas respond. Furthermore, perceptions of solutions to problems will be conditional, and constrained by political,

social and economic reality, limiting what can be attempted and what can be achieved (McKay and Cox 1978 p. 505).

In other words, public policy is likely to require complex explanation, that is, in terms of more than one theory (Klein 1974 pp. 219-220). Moreover, there is a sense in which the several theories operate at different levels, the macro level being represented by economic and demographic variables, and the micro level by the behaviour of individuals and small groups. The major question upon which this book focusses, the relationships between doctors, government and managers, is formulated at a third, meso (or middle), level, that is at the level of entire occupational groups within an entire policy sector. Thus, a change at this level, from 'ideological corporatism' to a challenge by the 'corporate rationalisers', has been explained by changes at the other two levels, with actors' 'assumptive worlds' providing, as it were, the links between levels.

This notion of levels of theoretical explanation has been the subject of a good deal of recent academic interest (Ham and Hill 1984; Pettigrew 1985; Cawson 1985; Alford and Friedland 1985), though there seems to be little consensus about how precisely it should be used in the analysis of specific circumstances (cf. Ham 1982 p. 164; 1985 pp. 196-197; Hambleton 1986 pp. 31-33). Moreover, it is not without its critics (Giddens 1984 p. 139; Saunders 1986 p. 311). Nevertheless, the present study has provided, at least, one instance of a policy shift which cannot be fully explained without resort to a variety of theories.

Chapter 7

1985 AND AFTER: SHIFTING THE FRONTIER?

This final chapter has three main purposes. Firstly, it considers how far the Griffiths and related reforms have succeeded in shifting the location of NHS managers in terms of Figure 1.2; that is, can they now be regarded as agents of government rather than facilitators for doctors? The conclusion reached, though on the basis of rather unsystematic evidence, is that they probably can. In Alford's (1975) terms, the managers are indeed the 'corporate rationalisers'. But this does not necessarily make them (still in Alford's terms) the dominant structural interest, and the second purpose of the chapter is therefore to consider how much of a shift has occurred in the 'frontier of control' between doctors and managers. The conclusion reached in this respect is that some change has taken place, but that this has been more to do with the form of relationships than with the substance. Thirdly, the chapter is concerned to assess future prospects, in the context both of what seem to be natural limits on the extent to which British governments might wish to restrict clinical freedom, and of further structural changes which might follow the Government's present review of funding arrangements for the NHS.

The conclusions on all these matters are, of course, subject to a number of caveats. Although Sir Roy Griffiths himself has said that noticeable impact would occur within three to five years of the managerial changes (Social Services Committee 1984 p. 141), it is still premature to be drawing firm conclusions, especially since a number of studies whose fieldwork was in progress at the time of the implementation of the post-1982 changes seem not to have detected any sudden change (Haywood and Ranade 1985 p. iii; Thompson 1986 p. 57; Long et al 1987 pp. 48-50). Moreoever, information about the funding options under consideration in the

Government review is sketchy in the extreme, and predictions are therefore difficult. Finally, the reader should note that this chapter is neither an assessment of the impact of the Griffiths changes as a whole (for which the outcome of a number of continuing studies will have to be awaited), nor an analysis of the impact upon staff other than managers and doctors (for a preliminary attempt at which, see Harrison 1988b).

One important issue upon which this book has otherwise been silent, the question of whether or not a shift in the frontier of control is desirable, is briefly addressed in a concluding comment to the Chapter.

MANAGERS AS AGENTS OF GOVERNMENT?

Evidence of change in the government-manager relationship is of two main kinds. Firstly, there is evidence that NHS managers are now under much more pressure than before (see Chapter 3) to comply with central government directives and priorities. One medium for this is the revised Review Process (see Chapter 4); officers of the NHS Management Board now meet directly with Regional General Managers, resulting, according to one member of the Board, in 'a marked change in regional behaviour' in the implementation of cost-improvement programmes (Mills 1987 p. 470). High-profile political initiatives, such as that concerning the reduction of hospital waiting lists (Moore 1987c) are another such medium, whilst statutory changes to make Family Practitioner Committees directly responsible to the DHSS (see Chapter 4) seem to have led to their officers seeing themselves less as local agents for independent contractors and more as agents of government (Allsop and May 1986 pp. 3-4; Anderson 1987c p. 922).

The second kind of available evidence relates to managers' apparent reluctance publicly to challenge anything emanating from the centre. Thus one health authority Chairman instructed his District's managers not to seek additional funding since 'the District must be seen to be on the side of the Region and the Secretary of State' (Health Service Journal 26 November 1987 p. 1366). In a different Region, the Regional General Manager declined to give evidence to a public enquiry into his Region's funding, saying

>It is not our job as health authorities to demand more money for the health service in the Region. It is the Government's job to allocate funds (Moore 1987a p. 464).

Considerable pressure has also been exerted upon doctors in management posts not to contest government policy, even to the point of suspension and dismissal (Health Service Journal 28 May 1987 p. 604; Observer 27 December 1987 p. 4). In such a climate, reports that DHSS has adopted a practice of censoring RHAs' press releases to make them 'more positive' came as no surprise (Alleway 1987b p. 348).

The evidence, then, is consistent with a picture of increasing central control over local managers, though it is important to note two qualifying comments. Firstly, it is almost certainly the managers at RHA level who are most vulnerable; given that they now run few services of their own, their raison d'etre has increasingly become the communication of government priorities to the rest of the NHS. Secondly, the increased central control seems to be at its strongest in particular domains: those which can be reported back to DHSS in quantitative or financial terms. It has proved much more difficult to enforce policies in less easily quantifiable areas such as the implementation of management budget systems (Pollitt et al 1988) or quality assurance (Shaw 1986).

SHIFTING THE FRONTIER?

How far have the Griffiths and related changes affected doctors? The medical profession can certainly be regarded as having suffered a number of defeats concerning the introduction of general management. The immediate response of the British Medical Association (BMA) to the publication of the Griffiths Report was to complain at the perceived lack of time for consultation, to challenge the concept of a non-medical general manager, to demand the retention of District Management Teams, and to seek the provision of an appeals mechanism against managers' decisions (British Medical Journal Vol. 287, 1983 pp. 1321-1322, 1643, 1811). It also sought, in place of the general manager proposed by

Griffiths, the election from within existing teams of a Chairman [sic], and a trial period for any changes adopted (Social Services Committee 1984 pp, 1-13; British Medical Journal Vol. 288, 1984 p. 84). It was further argued that management at the unit level of organisation was best left to doctors, and that the proposed Supervisory and Management Boards should include clinicians.

In the event, none of these preferences prevailed, and by 1984 the BMA's Annual Representatives Meeting was being told by one of its officials that 'management by managers' was here to stay (British Medical Journal Vol. 289, 1984 p. 201), although, ironically, offical sources were still assuring the profession that policy towards management teams had remained unchanged (British Medical Journal, Vol. 289, 1984 p. 1470). The medical profession was also defeated in terms of its penetration of general manager appointments (see above, Table 4.1), and of its demands for remuneration for participation in management budgets, and for budgetary accountability to be solely within the profession (British Medical Journal, Vol. 287, 1984 p. 1812), though payment for undertaking management duties was obtained (DHSS 1985d).

These defeats for the medical profession are, however, ones of form rather than substance. It does not follow that they will have any impact on the substance of doctor-manager relations; organisational formalities do not always have their intended effect (Blau 1955) and in any case can be used by managers in a variety of ways. Thus, for example, management budget systems could be used for a variety of purposes ranging from merely providing information to clinicians to imposing output targets upon them (Lamb and David 1985 p. 651). When it comes to an examination of the substance of manager-doctor relations, it is rather difficult to discern great change.

Indeed the major changes that have occurred have been restrictions in clinical freedom imposed by government, that is, a shift in the frontier of control, but not as a result of managers' efforts. Hence, restrictions on the growth of NHS resources (see Chapter 5), and the introduction of additional prescribing restrictions (see Chapter 4 and Bryan 1986) are probably much more significant than any managerial action. This is not to say that no managerial action has impinged on doctors. Ham's study of two District Health Authorities suggests that managers were sometimes able to override consultant interests in the formulation of local health policies (Ham 1986 p. 128). Similarly, a recent study of the use of Performance Indicators (the introduction of which was not challenged by the medical profession: Harrison 1988b) provides a number of examples of consultant influence being apparently diminished by the availability of management information (Jenkins et al 1987 pp. 83, 126-167). Other examples include the managerial imposition of restrictions upon General Practitioners' ability to refer to at least one London teaching hospital (Health Service Journal, 13 August 1987 p. 924), and what has been alleged in respect of one Region as a policy of suspending from duty doctors who publicly opposed spending cuts and bed closures (Yorkshire Post, 23 February 1988 p. 3).

Thus, despite the 1987 Annual Representatives Meeting of the BMA having felt it necessary to adopt the motion that doctors should be accountable to general managers only where the former had accepted managerial duties (Hildrew 1987 p. 2), there seems, post-Griffiths as pre-Griffiths, to have been relatively little doctor-manager conflict. Moreover, where such conflict has occurred, the medical profession has often been the winner. Thus, management budget systems have continued to hold only trial status (British Medical Journal Vol. 288, 1984 pp. 162, 165) since initial broad clinician support for the notion (Stewart 1984; Harrison et al 1984a) has narrowed to those who see budgetary information primarily as a vehicle to argue for additional resources (Pollitt et al 1988). Sir Roy Griffiths has found it necessary to assure doctors that general managers will not assess clinical performance (Health Service Journal, 11 December 1986 p. 1593), whilst General Practitioners have so far managed to resist DHSS proposals for a 'good practice' allowance (Tynedale 1987 p. 6, though see DHSS et al 1987 p. 16) and to weaken proposals for stricter controls of deputising services (DHSS 1984e p. 3). The profession has also succeeded in preventing general managers from attending Consultant selection interviews (Health Service Journal, 8 October 1987 p. 1153), and securing the reinstatement of a community physician suspended for publicly criticising economy measures (Johnson 1988

p. 3). Unresolved issues at the time of writing included a Scottish Health Board's reported attempt to plan medical manpower without adequately consulting clinicians (Moore 1987b p. 864; Health Service Journal, 28 March 1988 p. 323), and a Regional Health Authority's attempt to introduce more detailed contracts of employment for consultants (Anderson 1987a p. 777).

It is also easy to suggest initiatives which might have been taken but were not. A radical management approach might have been expected to question consultants' distinction awards, made at present within the profession on non-managerial criteria (Ludbrooke and Mooney 1984 p. 421). Similarly, the subject matter of Rayner Scrutinies (see above, Chapter 4) has been confined to matters unlikely to have adverse impact on doctors (DHSS 1982d; 1985e). They might, for instance, have included an examination of expenditure on junior doctors' overtime payments. Nor, apparently, has the successful development of computer-aided diagnosis (Adams et al 1986 p. 80ff) led to any central attempt to diffuse it more widely.

To summarise: although NHS managers are more clearly agents of government than before, and although the frontier of control between government and doctors has shifted a little, in favour of the former, there is as yet little evidence that managers have secured greater control over doctors. It should be restated that this is an early conclusion, based on scant and unsystematic evidence of the sort exemplified earlier in this section; one current matter which will perhaps provide the acid test of whether managers can implement policy against the interests of consultant medical staff is Achieving a Balance (British Medical Journal, Vol. 293, 1986 pp. 147-151). If the plans for medical manpower and career arrangements contained in this document are successfully implemented, they will mark the end of two decades of medical resistance to a substantial increase in the ratio of consultants to junior hospital doctors, and to the introduction of a permanent sub-consultant career grade. (For a review, see Long et al 1987 pp. 62-67).

This apparent relative lack of impact of the Griffiths and related changes can be explained, using the theoretical material discussed in earlier Chapters, in terms of three observations, one relating to the medical profession itself, the second to NHS managers, and the third to govern- ments. Taken together, these observations show why the ostensible challenge to doctors of recent innovations in management has not been sustained.

Firstly, despite the limitations on overall finan- cial resources for the NHS, and the consequent sharpening of the rationing debate, the basic sources of (in Alford's terms) the doctors' struc- tural monopoly remain unchanged. It is still general practitioners who provide the selection of cases for consultants to work upon. It is still consultants who decide which, and how many, patients to see, how to diagnose and treat them, when to admit and when to discharge them. It is still not possible for health authority managers to ensure that they recruit consultants whose clinical interests match local priorities, and most consul- tants are employed by Regional Health Authorities rather than by the District Health Authorities in whose premises and upon whose residents they practise. The prime determinant of the pattern of health services is still, just as before Griffiths, what doctors choose to do.

Secondly, there are serious limits to the nature of the control which NHS managers, in the present system of health care in Britain, might seek over doctors. These limits arise from the (for managers) complexity and unpredictability of medical work; as the theories of Lindblom and Simon discussed in Chapter 6 suggest, managers simply cannot plan and control everything. This is compounded by the principle that care is supposed to be individualised for particular patients. The point has been made succinctly by Lipsky in his more general discussion of the role of 'street-level bureaucrats', that is, public service professionals such as doctors, teachers and social workers. Because demands for the time of such workers exceed its supply, they are left to devise simplifying decision rules in order to process clients; hence

.....the decisions of street-level bureaucrats, the routines they establish, and the devices they invent to cope with uncertainties and work pressures, effectively become the public policies they carry out (Lipsky 1980 p. xii, emphasis original.)

Moreover, because performance measurement in health
care is difficult to define and often ambiguous
(see, for instance, Pollitt's critiques of
Performance Indicators: Pollitt 1985a; 1985b; 1986),
managerial systems find it elusive to control.
Professional 'clan' culture may be more effective;

> Behaviour within the clan is regulated through
> mutual monitoring by.... members, utilising....
> norms not susceptible to exact translation into
> performance measures. Clinical freedom is....
> a form of clan control.... It minimises
> [management] costs for an organisation such as
> the NHS which is characterised by high ambi-
> guity of performance measures and relatively
> high agreement about operational objectives
> (Bourn and Ezzamel 1986 pp. 206, 213; see also
> Majone 1986 pp. 451, 454).

There is, of course, evidence from the pre-Griffiths
NHS (see above, Chapter 3), that such complexity
breeds frustration on the part of managers. But one
of the things which the Griffiths and related
changes have done, is to give managers greater control over non-medical groups of staff (Confederation
of Health Service Employees 1987; Harrison 1988b),
and perhaps thereby to reduce such frustration.
Certainly recent evidence given to the Social
Services Committee on behalf of managers suggests a
greater degree of contentment than before (Institute
of Health Services Management, 1987 p. 3), and it
would not be surprising if NHS managers were somewhat reluctant to seek conflict with doctors. The
disproportionately high attrition rate of general
managers appointed from outside the NHS (see above,
Table 4.1) may well stand as testimony to the
inadvisability of such conflict (see, for instance,
Health Service Journal, 4 February 1988 p. 136).

Thirdly, marxist theory serves to remind that it is
not only doctors who benefit from the operation of
clinical freedom, though much sociological (see, for
instance, Johnson 1972 pp. 42-43) and medical criticism of the notion has focussed upon it as a means
by which doctors avoid control and accountability:

> [The doctor] can see whatever patients consult
> him; he can give whatever advice he pleases,
> however unorthodox, and provide whatever
> treatment he pleases, however expensive or
> lethal; he can behave towards his patients

however he pleases and extract from them
whatever they will pay (Fox, quoted in Smith
1987, p. 1583).

But clinical freedom is also a device by which decisions about how to ration medical care are rendered
invisible:

> By various means, physicians.... try to make
> the denial of care seem routine or optimal.
> Confronted by a person older than the
> prevailing unofficial age of cut-off for
> dialysis, the British GP tells the victim of
> chronic renal failure or his family that
> nothing can be done except to make the patient
> as comfortable as possible in the time
> remaining. The British nephrologist tells the
> family of a patient who is difficult to handle
> that dialysis would be painful and burdensome
> and that the patient would be more comfortable
> without it (Aaron and Schwartz 1984 p. 101).

The point is that, because such decisions are
individual and fragmented, the reality of rationing
is not publicly evident. It is, of course, governments (and health service managers) who are thereby
spared decisions which would be politically almost
impossible in a health service which purports to be
comprehensive. From such a perspective, the government's managerial and efficiency strategy for the
NHS has already served its purpose by legitimising
expenditure restrictions. The solution is a symbolic one (Pfeffer and Salancik 1978 pp. 263-266;
Elder and Cobb 1983 pp. 18-21), and requires only
that doctors do not persistently and publicly
challenge it.

THE FUTURE: TWO SCENARIOS

It follows from all this that, unless there are
major structural changes in the NHS, the future for
the frontier of control will not be much different
from the present. But structural changes may well
be on the political agenda, for the Government is
reported to be conducting a further review into the
funding of health care in Britain (Timmins and Brown
1987 p. 13, Brown and Timmins 1988 p. 5).

This seems to have been a response to demands for
additional NHS funding, as manifest in a number of

incidents such as the repeated postponement by a
health authority of surgery for a hole-in-the-heart
baby (Yorkshire Post, 30 November 1987 p. 3) and
direct approaches to the Prime Minister by the
Central Committee for Hospital Medical Services (an
officially recognised doctors' representative body)
and the presidents of the three Royal Colleges,
of Physicians, Surgeons and Obstetricians and
Gynaecologists (Millar 1987b p. 1426). A number of
Conservative MPs, including a former Minister for
Health, have also been arguing to the same end
(Anderson 1987b p. 1395).

According to press reports, the review is
considering (presumably in addition to the retention
of the status quo) three broad options for the
future, all involving some degree of additional use
of the market (Timmins 1988; Oakley and Wood 1988).
The least radical of these options seems to be along
lines originally proposed by Enthoven (1985), in
which District Health Authorities would each be
responsible for paying for the care of their
resident populations, irrespective of where such
care was actually provided; this would entail cross-
charging, in place of the present system of
retrospective adjustments of RAWP revenue targets,
for patients treated in another District. Other
options, as will be seen below, are more radical.

The possible future for the frontier of control
between doctors and managers can therefore be seen
in terms of two broad scenarios; a conservative
scenario in which the status quo is either retained,
or modified by the introduction of cross-charging
between District Health Authorities, and a radical
scenario in which more fundamental structural
changes are made. Each of these is discussed in
turn.

Even the conservative scenario entails some further
breaches of clinical freedom. If cross-charging
were introduced, GPs' referral rights would have to
be curtailed, since otherwise a health authority
would not be able to manage its expenditure. But
such restrictions are, as noted above, already
beginning to creep into the service. There is
evidence that doctors tend to use the notion of
clinical freedom as a rhetorical tool; that is, they
employ it defensively when threatened by developments which, if subsequently adopted, they quickly
rationalise and cease to regard as a breach of

clinical freedom (Harrison et al 1984b). If this evidence can be generalised (and experience with prescribing restrictions suggests that it might well be), then referral restrictions will be accepted with relatively little conflict. Similarly, hospital doctors are likely to find themselves under even greater pressure to be cost-conscious than at present, especially if, as has been suggested, such services as Pathology are made the subject of competitive tendering (Independent, 13 January 1988 p. 6).

But none of these changes suggest major modifications in clinicians' behaviour; cross-boundary flow represents a minority of patients, and privatised pathology contracts, given a high ratio of fixed to variable costs, would necessarily have to specify in advance a volume of tests to be conducted. In the conservative scenario, there seems little reason for health authorities to engage in more than marginally competitive behaviour. In such a scenario, the prime managerial strategy towards doctors is likely to be co-optation of the latter into managerial ways of thinking and acting, rather than direct attempts at control. As the best-selling text In Search of Excellence notes, albeit in a commercial context,

....the stronger the culture and the more it was directed toward the marketplace, the less need was there for policy manuals, organisational charts, or detailed procedures and rules ....[P]eople way down the line know what they are supposed to do in most situations because the handful of guiding values is crystal clear (Peters and Waterman 1982 pp. 75-76).

Such an approach - changing the organisational culture of the NHS - follows logically from the Griffiths Report's enjoinder that clinicians should be more closely involved in the management process (NHS Management Inquiry 1983 p. 6). Indeed, a number of commentators have made such an approach the centrepiece of their prescription for change in the NHS (see, for instance, Health Services Management Centre 1984), and it has found practical application in national strategies to appoint doctors as general managers (see above, Chapter 4), and for the provision of management education for clinicians (National Health Service Training Authority 1986). According to early studies of

general management, it is also manifest in the local
management strategies adopted by general managers
(Stewart et al 1987 pp. 7-11; Scrivens 1987 p. 17
ff). In summary, then, the conservative scenario
envisages a slow shift in the frontier of control,
accompanied by an increasing tendency on the part of
doctors themselves to think in managerial,
especially cost, terms.

The radical scenario is derived from two other
health sevice funding options said to be under government consideration (Timmins 1988). Both imply
the fragmentation of present NHS authorities into
smaller units, for whom successful competition would
be a precondition for survival. One option is said
to be the funding of health care through an identi-
fiable national insurance contribution, rather than
as at present mainly through general taxation, thus
allowing members of the public to opt out of the NHS
in favour of private care. Hospitals and other
health care insitutions might also be able to opt
out of the NHS and to compete for patients (see, for
instance, Brittan 1988). The other option which
constitutes the radical scenario is movement in the
direction of Health Maintenance Organisations
(HMOs), as currently found in the United States.
(For a basic, though partisan, account see Butler
1987). Under such an arrangement public and private
health care institutions would compete to offer
pre-paid health care cover to the public, with a
basic level of premium met by the government, perhaps in the form of a voucher, but with the option
for subscribers to purchase additional levels of
cover.

In such a scenario, price competition between
institutions is likely to be crucial, and doctors
are therefore likely to be placed under much more
specific management pressures than in the conservative scenario to control the level of costs
incurred in treating particular patients, and to
show that they are contributing to the 'earnings' of
their employer. This will certainly result in the
abandonment of the quasi-ownership of hospital beds
by individual clinicians, and, if American experience is any guide, the development of management-
imposed controls such as standardised diagnostic and
treatment protocols (Richards 1986; Butler 1987 p.
296), seen by clinicians as a reduction in their
clinical freedom (Schulz and Scheckler, 1988 pp.
8,11). In terms of Alford's theory of structural

128

interests, the 'corporate rationalisers' would become the dominant interest.

Implementation of the radical scenario would represent a failure of the Government's management and efficiency strategy for the NHS as conducted to date; that is, it would show that the Griffiths and related reforms had failed to stem demands for additional public expenditure on health care, and that clinical freedom could no longer be relied upon to ration health care unobtrusively. The radical scenario would thus be the logical solution to a renewed government dilemma of how to maintain economic policy in the face of demands for additional health care expenditure. As many earlier radical right-wing prescriptions for the NHS have suggested, the use of markets is likely to stimulate additional expenditure, but from private sources (see, for instance, Adam Smith Institute n.d. p. 7; Seldon 1980 p. 145).

These, then, are the broad possible futures for the manager-doctor relationship in British health care. That the radical scenario will actually come about is far from certain. It would probably be costly in government and parliamentary time, and would probably destroy what is often considered in government circles to be an excellent relationship between DHSS and the medical profession. Moreover, it is still possible that ad hoc injections of additional funds (Timmins and Brown 1987 p. 1) and full funding of NHS staff pay awards (Anderson 1988 p. 227) will be sufficient to stem expenditure demands. And there is little obviously radical in the proposals related to GPs in the recent white paper Promoting Better Health (DHSS et al 1987 pp. 11-24). But the frontier of control is currently more unstable than ever before in the history of the NHS.

A CONCLUDING COMMENT

One question which this book has not addressed merits a concluding comment. This concerns a value judgement as to whether or not any shift in the frontier of control is desirable.

The medical profession has always preferred to travel hopefully rather than to arrive. ....If investigation and treatment are to be limited, we must know which investigations and which treatments are valuable and which are not.... Clinical freedom died accidentally, crushed between the rising costs of new forms of investigation and treatment and the financial limits inevitable in an economy that cannot expand indefinitely. Clinical freedom should, however, have been strangled long ago ... We must welcome its demise and seize the opportunities now laid out before us (Hampton 1983 pp. 1237-1238).

The above words were written by a Professor of Cardiology and published in the British Medical Journal. If he is right that clinical freedom is dead (and it has been argued above that it is by no means certain that it is) then is he justified in welcoming its demise? Such a justification must rest on the reasoning that less freedom will in some sense produce benefits for patients, and indeed Hampton's message is to doctors: to evaluate their care and treatment practices. But this cannot be equated with a conclusion that greater governmental or managerial control over doctors will produce the same results. It is simply not self-evident that shifting the frontier of control between doctors and third parties will produce such an effect; in Alford's terms the consumers may still be repressed. In particular, those developments aimed at producing 'better performance' in the NHS risk the stimulation of a whole range of perverse behaviours aimed at circumventing the evaluation system (see, for instance, Times, 14 October 1986 p. 7).

To be crudely in favour of, or against, the managerial reforms which are the subject of this book is to disregard this crucial observation. No mechanism can guarantee the appropriate behaviour by doctors, but Hampton may well be right; more extensive and active peer review and audit arrangements (something which has recently been proposed for general practice; DHSS et al 1987 pp. 16, 23) within the medical profession would represent a scenario more desirable than any other organisational changes within the NHS.

REFERENCES

Aaron, H.J. & Schwartz W.B. (1984) The Painful
    Prescription: Rationing Hospital Care,
    Washington D.C., Brookings Institution
Abel-Smith, B. (1967) 'Administrative Solution: A
    Hospital Commissioner?' in B. Robb (ed.), Sans
    Everything: A Case to Answer, London, Nelson
Adams, I.D., Chan, M., Clifford, P.C., Cooke, W.M.,
    Dallos, V., de Dombal, F.T., Edwards, M.H.,
    Hancock, D.M., Hewett, D.J., McIntyre, N.,
    Somerville, P.G., Speigelhalter, D.J.,
    Wellwood, J. & Wilson, D.H. (1986) 'Computer-
    Aided Diagnosis of Acute Abdominal Pain: A
    Multicentre Study', British Medical Journal,
    Vol. 293, pp. 800-804
Adam Smith Institute (n.d.), Health and the Public
    Sector: A Report to the Minister of Health,
    London
Advisory Commitee for Management Efficiency in the
    National Health Service (1966) Management
    Functions of Hospital Doctors, London, Ministry
    of Health
Alexander, A. (1982) Local Government in Britain
    Since Reorganisation, London, Allen and Unwin
Alford, R.R. (1975) Health Care Politics, Chicago,
    Ill., University of Chicago Press
Alford, R.R. & Friedland, R. (1985) Powers of
    Theory: Capitalism, the State, and Democracy,
    Cambridge, Cambridge University Press
Allen, D.E. (1979) Hospital Planning: the
    Development of the 1962 Hospital Plan,
    Tunbridge Wells, Pitman Medical
Alleway, L. (1987a) 'A Very Sweet Secret
    Secretariat', Health Service Journal, 2 July,
    pp. 762-763
Alleway, L. (1987b) 'DHSS Admits Censoring RHA Press
    Releases', Health Service Journal, 26 March, p.
    348
Alleway, L. & Anderson, F. (1986) 'Health Education
    Council to Reform to Tackle AIDS', Health
    Service Journal, 27 November, p. 1531
Allsop, J. (1984) Health Policy and the National
    Health Service, London, Longmans
Allsop, J. & May A. (1986) The Emperor's New
    Clothes: Family Practitioner Committees in the
    1980s, London, King Edward's Hospital Fund for
    London
Anderson, F. (1987a) 'South-Western Managers
    "Insensitive and Alienating"', Health Service
    Journal, 9 July, p. 777

131

REFERENCES

Anderson, F. (1987b) 'Former Health Minister Attacks Underfunding', Health Service Journal, Vol. 97, p. 1395

Anderson, F. (1987c) 'FPC Agrees to Undergo Appraisal by Mersey Region', Health Service Journal, 13 August, p. 922

Anderson, F. (1988) 'Newton Hints at Funding of Review Body Awards', Health Service Journal, 25 February, p. 227

Arthur Young (1986a) Practical Management Budgeting in the NHS: A New Initiative for Successful Implementation, Glasgow

Arthur Young (1986b) Evaluating Management Budgeting in the NHS: A Practical Guide, Glasgow

Ascher, K. (1987) The Politics of Privatisation: Contracting Out Public Services, London, Macmillan

Baines, P. (1985) 'History and Rationale of the 1979 Reforms' in G. Drewry (ed.), The New Select Committees: A Study of the 1979 Reforms, pp. 13-36, Oxford, Clarendon Press

Barber, W.J. (1967) A History of Economic Thought, Harmondsworth, Pelican

Barnard, K. & Harrison, S. (1984) 'Memorandum' in Social Services Committee, First Report Session 1983-84: Griffiths NHS Management Inquiry Report, HC 209, London, House of Commons/HMSO

Barnard, K. & Harrison S. (1986) 'Labour Relations in Health Services Management', Social Science and Medicine, Vol. 22, no. 11, pp. 1213-1228

Barnard, K., Lee, K., Mills, A. & Reynolds, J. (1979) Towards a New Rationality: a Study of Planning in the NHS (in four volumes), Leeds, University of Leeds, Nuffield Centre for Health Services Studies

Barnard, K., Lee, K., Mills, A. & Reynolds, J. (1980) 'NHS Planning: an Assessment', Hospital and Health Services Review, Vol. 76, nos. 8 & 9, pp. 262-265, 301-304

Blau, P.M. (1955) The Dynamics of Bureaucracy, Chicago, Ill., University of Chicago Press

Bosanquet, N. (ed.) 1979 Industrial Relations in the NHS: the Search for a System, London, King's Fund

Bourn, M. & Ezzamel, M. (1986) 'Organisational Culture in Hospitals in the National Health Service', Financial Accountability and Management, Vol. 2, no. 3, pp. 203-225

Brittan, L. (1988) A New Deal for Health Care, London, Conservative Political Centre

REFERENCES

Brown, C. & Timmins (1988) 'Support Group Will Aid
    Health Review', The Independent, 5 February,
    p. 5
Brown, R.G.S. (1979) Reorganising the National
    Health Service: A Case Study of Administrative
    Change, Oxford, Blackwell and Martin Robertson
Brown, R.G.S., Griffin, S. & Haywood, S.C. (1975)
    New Bottles: Old Wine?, Hull, University of
    Hull, Institute for Health Studies
Bryan, J. (1986) 'First Birthday for the Limited
    List', Health Service Journal, 27 March, p. 426
Buckland, R. (1987) 'The Costs and Returns of the
    Privatisation of Nationalised Industries',
    Public Administration, Vol. 65, no. 3, pp. 241-
    257
Butler, E. (1987) 'HMOs - A New Management Model
    from the United States', Journal of Management
    in Medicine, Vol. 1, no. 4, pp. 290-299
Carvel, J. & Perera S. (1988) 'Newton Pledge on
    Nursing Pay Cut', Guardian, 9 January, p. 30
Cawson, A. (1985) 'Varieties of Corporatism: the
    importance of the meso-level of interest
    intermediation' in A. Caswon (ed.), Organised
    Interests and the State: Studies in Meso-
    Corporatism, London, Sage
CBI Working Party on Government Expenditure (1981)
    Report, London, Confederation of British
    Industry
Central Health Services Council (1954) (Chairman:
    Alderman A.F. Bradbeer) Report of the Committee
    on the Internal Administration of Hospitals,
    London, HMSO
Central Policy Review Staff (1975) A Joint Framework
    for Social Policies, London, HMSO
Central Statistical Office (1983) Annual Abstract of
    Statistics, London, HMSO
Central Statistical Office (1986) Social Trends 16,
    London, HMSO
Chaplin, N.W. (ed.) (1987) The Hospitals and Health
    Services Yearbook and Directory of Hospital
    Suppliers, London, Institute of Health Services
    Management
Charlton, J.R.H., Silver, R., Hartley, R.M. &
    Holland, W.W. (1983) 'Geographical Variations
    in Mortality from Conditions Amenable to
    Medical Intervention in England and Wales', The
    Lancet, 25 March
Cohen, M.D., March, J.G. & Olsen, J.P. (1972) 'A
    Garbage Can Model of Organisational Choice',
    Administrative Science Quarterly, Vol. 72, no.
    1, pp. 1-25

REFERENCES

Committee of Enquiry into the Cost of the National
Health Service (1956) (Chairman: Mr C.W.
Guillebaud) Report, Cmnd 663, London, HMSO
Committee of Enquiry into Allegations of Ill-
Treatment of Patients and Other Irregularities
at Ely Hospital, Cardiff (1969) (Chairman: Mr
Geoffrey Howe) Report, London, HMSO
Committee of Inquiry into Normansfield Hospital
(1978) (Chairman: Mr M.D. Sherrard) Report,
Cmnd 7357, London, HMSO
Committee of Public Accounts (1981) Seventh Report,
Session 1980-81: Financial Control and
Accountability in the National Health Sevice,
London, House of Commons/HMSO
Committee of Public Accounts (1982) Seventh Report,
Session 1981-82: Financial Control and
Accountability in the National Health Service;
Cost of Remedying Defects in Hospitals; Working
Practices in the National Health Service,
London, House of Commons/HMSO
Committee of Public Accounts (1984) Sixteenth
Report, Session 1983-84: Manpower Control,
Accountability and Other Matters Relating to
the National Health Service, London, House of
Commons/HMSO
Committee of Public Accounts (1986) Forty-Second
Report, Session 1985-86: Value for Money
Developments in the National Health Service;
Energy Conservation, London, House of
Commons/HMSO
Committee on the Civil Service (1968) (Chairman:
Lord Fulton) Report, Cmnd 3638, London, HMSO
Confederation of Health Service Employees (1987)
Final Report: The Impact of General Management
and General Managers in the NHS, Banstead
Conservative Party (1979), Election Manifesto, April
Conservative Party (1987) Our First Eight Years: The
Achievements of the Conservative Government
Since May 1979, London
Council for Science & Society (1982) Expensive
Medical Techniques, London
Cyert, R.M. & March, J.G. (1963) A Behavioural
Theory of the Firm, Englewood Cliffs, N.J.,
Prentice-Hall
Dalton, M. (1959) Men Who Manage, New York, Wiley
Davidson, N. (1983) 'Alliance to Top Slice £500
million', Health and Social Service Journal, 2
June, pp. 650-651

REFERENCES

Davies, G. & Piachaud, D. (1985) 'Public Expenditure
     and the Social Services: The Economic and
     Political Constraints' in R.E. Klein and M.
     O'Higgins (eds), The Future of Welfare, Oxford,
     Blackwell
Davies, P. (1985) 'Public Accounts Committee: the
     Lion's Den for Accounting Offices', Health
     Service Journal, 7 November, pp. 1398-1399
Davies, P. (1986a) 'The Day the Chairman Left',
     Health Sevice Journal, 12 June, p. 784
Davies, P. (1986b) 'Counting the Cost of Cuts',
     Health Service Journal, 26 June, pp. 850-851
Davies, P. (1986c) 'Agnostic Over Grifftiths',
     Health Service Journal, 12 June, p. 785
Davies, P. (1987) 'The Public Voices its Opinions on
     the NHS', Health Service Journal, 2 April, pp.
     382-383
Day, P. & Klein, R.E. (1983) 'The Mobilisation of
     Consent versus the Management of Conflict:
     Decoding the Griffiths Report', British Medical
     Journal, Vol. 287, pp. 1813-1815
Department of Health & Social Security (1970) The
     Future Structure of the National Health
     Service (The Crossman Green Paper), London,
     HMSO
Department of Health & Social Security (1972a)
     National Health Service Reorganisation:
     England, Cmnd 5055, London, HMSO
Department of Health & Social Security (1972b)
     Management Arrangements for the Reorganised
     National Health Service, London, HMSO
Department of Health & Social Security (1976) The
     NHS Planning System, London
Department of Health & Social Security (1979a)
     'Patrick Jenkin: the Royal Commission and
     Pharmacy', Press Release no. 79/216, 11
     September
Department of Health & Social Security (1979b) 'The
     NHS and the Future: Sound Economy the Key',
     Press Release no. 79/153, 20 June
Department of Health & Social Security (1979c)
     '"Waiting Lists Could be Cut in Two" Says Dr
     Gerard Vaughan', Press Release no. 79/237, 27
     September
Department of Health & Social Security (1979d)
     'Patients Before Bureaucrats: Patrick Jenkin on
     his Plans for the NHS', Press Release no.
     79/322, 14 December
Department of Health & Social Security (1979e)
     'Health Service Cash Limits: Mr Jenkin's
     Speech', Press Release no. 79/183, 18 July

REFERENCES

Department of Health & Social Security (1979f)
    'Local Management, Not Centralised Bureaucracy:
    Mr Patrick Jenkin Indentifies the Needs of the
    NHS', Press Release no. 79/133, 30 May
Department of Health & Social Security (1980a) 'NHS
    Information and Statistical Services to be
    Revised: Steering Group Set Up', Press Release
    no. 80/29, 7 February
Department of Health & Social Security (1980b)
    Health Service Development: Structure and
    Management, Circular HC(80)8
Department of Health & Social Security (1980c)
    'Patrick Jenkin Firmly Rejects Committee's
    Strictures: Committee Failed to Ask the Right
    Questions', Press Release no. 80/302, 2
    December
Department of Health & Social Security (1980d)
    'Statement on Lambeth, Southwark and Lewisham
    Health Authority', Press Release no. 80/52, 3
    March
Department of Health & Social Security (1981a)
    'Consultants' Contracts: Mr Fowler's Decision',
    Press Release no. 81/260, 13 October
Department of Health & Social Security (1981b)
    'Money for NHS Increased 55% in Two Years: Dr
    Vaughan', Press Release no. 81/91, 3 April
Department of Health & Social Security (1982a) 'NHS
    to be Asked to Improve Accountability: Norman
    Fowler Announces New Moves and Regional
    Allocations', Press Release no. 82/14, 22
    January
Department of Health & Social Security (1982b)
    'Norman Fowler Announces New Moves on
    Efficiency', Press Release no 82/65, 11 March
Department of Health & Social Security (1982c) 'New
    Look at NHS Performance: Sir Derek Rayner to
    Advise on Scrutinies', Press Release no. 82/90,
    1 April
Department of Health & Social Security (1982d) 'Nine
    More Rayner Scrutinies in NHS', Press Release
    no. 82/240, 30 July
Department of Health & Social Security (1982e)
    'Working Group to Review Audit of NHS', Press
    Release no. 82/269, 27 August
Department of Health & Social Security (1982f)
    'Consultants to Review Control of Spending of
    Family Practitioner Services', Press Release
    82/306, 7 October

REFERENCES

Department of Health & Social Security (1983a)
'First National Package of Performance
Indicators for the NHS', Press Release no.
83/181, 22 September
Department of Health & Social Security (1983b)
Underused and Surplus Property in the National
Health Service: Report of the Enquiry Team
(Chairman: Mr Ceri Davies), London, HMSO
Department of Health & Social Security (1983c)
'Health Authorities to Review Their Property
Holdings', Press Release no. 83/257, 24
November
Department of Health & Social Security (1983d)
'Report Recommends Improvement to NHS Audit',
Press Release no. 83/156, 11 August
Department of Health & Social Security (1983e) 'NHS
Manpower Increase is Lowest Percentage since
1974: Norman Fowler', Press Release no. 83/12,
19 January
Department of Health & Social Security (1983f) 'More
Effective Prescribing of Pharmaceuticals',
Press Release no. 83/29, 4 February
Department of Health & Social Security (1983g)
Health Services Management: Competitive
Tendering in the Provision of Domestic,
Catering and Laundry Services, Circular
HC(83)18
Department of Health & Social Security (1983h)
'Tighter Controls on Deputising Services',
Press Release 83/287, 19 December
Department of Health & Social Security (1983i) 'NHS
Management Inquiry', Press Release no. 83/30, 3
February
Department of Health & Social Security (1983j) NHS
Management Inquiry, Circular no. DA(83)38
Department of Health & Social Security (1983k) 'The
NHS in a Changing World', Press Release no.
83/173, 12 September
Department of Health & Social Security (1983l) 'No
Government Plans to Change Financial Basis of
the NHS: Norman Fowler', Press Release no.
82/241, 30 July
Department of Health & Social Security (1983m)
Health Care and Its Costs: the Development of
the National Health Service in England, London,
HMSO
Department of Health & Social Security (1983n)
'Kenneth Clarke Asks FPCs to Check up on
Deputising Services', Press Release no. 83/139,
26 July

137

REFERENCES

Department of Health & Social Security (1984a)
    'Clarke on Limited List of Medicines', Press
    Release no. 84/360, 14 November
Department of Health & Social Security (1984b)
    'Griffiths Report - Health Authorities to
    Identify General Managers', Press Release no.
    84/173, 4 June
Department of Health & Social Security (1984c)
    'Chief Nursing Officer to Join NHS Supervisory
    Board: Norman Fowler', Press Release no. 84/138
Department of Health & Social Security (1984d)
    'Appointment of Chairman of the NHS Management
    Board', Press Release no. 84/418, 13 December
Department of Health & Social Security (1984e)
    'Deputising Services in General Medical
    Practice: Kenneth Clarke's Announcement', Press
    Release no. 84/71, 15 March
Department of Health & Social Security (1985a)
    'Performance Indicators for the NHS', Letter
    no. DA(85)19, 19 July
Department of Health & Social Security (1985b)
    Health Services Management: Management
    Budgeting, Circular HN(85)3
Department of Health & Social Security (1985c)
    'Health Service Plans for 1985/86: The Benefits
    to Patients', Press Release no. 85/109, 25
    April
Department of Health & Social Security (1985d)
    Health Services Management: Consultants and
    General Practitioners in General Management:
    Unit Medical Representatives with General
    Management Duties, Circular HC(85)9
Department of Health & Social Security (1985e) 'More
    Efficiency Scrutinies in the NHS', Press
    Release 85/352, 13 December
Department of Health & Social Security (1986a) 'NHS
    Management Board Appointments', Press Release
    no. 86/310, 2 October
Department of Health & Social Security (1986b)
    'Chairmanship of NHS Management Board', Press
    Release no. 86/174, 3 June
Department of Health & Social Security (1986c)
    Individual Performance Review, Circular no.
    PM(86)10
Department of Health & Social Security (1986d)
    General Managers: Arrangements for the
    Introduction of Performance-Related Pay,
    Circlar no. PM(86)11

REFERENCES

Department of Health & Social Security (1986e)
   Health Services Management: Resource Management
   (Management Budgeting) in Health Authorities,
   Circular HN(86)34
Department of Health & Social Security (1987) Health
   and Personal Social Services Statistics for
   England: 1987 Edition, London, HMSO
Department of Health & Social Security and Welsh
   Office (1979) Patients First: Consultative
   Paper on the Structure and Management of the
   National Health Service in England and Wales,
   London, HMSO
Department of Health & Social Security, Welsh
   Office, Northern Ireland Office & Scottish
   Office (1987) Promoting Better Health: the
   Government's Programme for Improving Primary
   Health Care, London, HMSO
Drewry, G. (ed.) (1985) The New Select Committees: A
   Study of the 1979 Reforms, Oxford, Clarendon
   Press
Drucker, P. (1979) Management, London, Pan Books
Dunleavy, P. (1981) 'Professions and Policy Change:
   Notes Towards a Model of Ideological
   Corporatism', Public Administration Bulletin,
   no. 36, pp. 3-16
Dunleavy, P. & O'Leary, B. (1987) Theories of the
   State: The Politics of Liberal Democracy,
   London, Macmillan
Eckstein, H. (1958) The English Health Service,
   Cambridge, Mass., Harvard University Press
Eckstein, H. (1960) Pressure Group Politics: the
   Case of the British Medical Association,
   London, Allen and Unwin
Elcock, H. & Haywood, S. (1980) The Buck Stops
   Where? Accountability and Control in the
   National Health Service, Hull, University of
   Hull, Institute for Health Studies
Elder, C.D. & Cobb, R.W. (1983) The Political Uses
   of Symbols, New York, Longmans
Elster, J. (1978) Logic and Society: Contradictions
   and Possible Worlds, Chichester, Wiley
Enthoven, A.C. (1985) Reflections on the Management
   of the National Health Service: an American
   looks at incentives to efficiency in health
   services management in the UK, London, Nuffield
   Provincial Hospitals Trust
Etzioni, A. (1967) 'Mixed-Scanning: A Third Approach
   to Decisionmaking', Public Administration
   Review, Vol. 27, pp. 385-392

REFERENCES

Fairey, M.J. (1985) 'Disc-Based Indicators', British
     Journal of Healthcare Computing, September, pp.
     9-10
Fairey, M.J., Condon, C., Darby, N., Donaldson, I.,
     Kenny, D. & Wickings I. (1975) A Review of the
     Management of the Reorganised NHS, London,
     Association of Chief Administrators of Health
     Authorities
Fayol, H. (1971) 'General Industrial Management',
     reprinted in D.S. Pugh (ed.), Organisational
     Theory, Harmondsworth, Penguin Books
Forsyth, G. (1966) Doctors and State Medicine: A
     Study of the British National Health Service,
     London, Pitman Medical
Forte, P.G.L. (1986) Decision-Making and Planning in
     a District Health Authority: A Review and a
     Case Study: Working Paper no. 466, Leeds,
     University of Leeds School of Geography
Fowler, N. (1982) Speech to Conservative Pary
     Conference, 6 October, Issued in Conservative
     Party News, Release no. 640/82
Fowler, N. (1983) Speech to National Association of
     Health Authorities, 24 June, Enclosed with
     Press Release no. 83/114
Fox, A. (1966) Industrial Sociology and Industrial
     Relations, Royal Commission on Trade Union and
     Employers' Associations, Research Paper no. 3,
     London, HMSO
Fredman, S. & Morris, G. (1987) 'The Teachers'
     Lesson: Collective Bargaining and the Courts',
     Industrial Law Journal, Vol. 16, no. 4, pp.
     215-226
Fry, G.K. (1984) 'The Development of the Thatcher
     Government's "Grand Strategy" for the Civil
     Service: a Public Policy Perspective', Public
     Administration, Vol. 62, pp. 322-335
Gamble, A.M. & Walkland, S.A. (1984) The British
     Party System and Economic Policy 1945-1983,
     Oxford, Clarendon Press
Garrett, J. (1986) 'Developing State Audit in
     Britain', Public Administration, Vol. 64, no.
     4, pp. 421-433
Giddens, A. (1984) The Constitution of Society:
     Outline of the Theory of Structuration,
     Cambridge, Polity Press
Giddings, P. (1985) 'What has been Achieved?' in G.
     Drewery (ed.), The New Select Committees: A
     Study of the 1979 Reforms, pp. 369-381, Oxford,
     Clarendon Press

REFERENCES

Gillion, C. & Hemming, R. (1985) 'Social Expenditure in the United Kingdom in a Comparative Context: Trends, Explanations and Projections' in R.E. Klein and M. O'Higgins (eds) The Future of Welfare, Oxford, Blackwell

Glennerster, H. (1985) Paying for Welfare, Oxford, Blackwell

Glennerster, H., Korman, N. & Marslen-Wilson, F. (1983) 'Plans and Practice: the Participants' Views', Public Administration, Vol. 61, no. 3, pp. 253-264

Goodrich, C.L. (1975) The Frontier of Control: a Study in British Workshop Politics, London, Pluto Press

Gough, I. (1979) The Political Economy of the Welfare State, London, Macmillan

Gray, A. & Jenkins, W.I. (1984) 'Lasting Reforms in Civil Service Management?', Political Quarterly, Vol. 55, pp. 418-427

Hallas, J. (1976) CHCs in Action, London, Nuffield Provincial Hospitals Trust

Halpern, S. (1983) 'The Quality Quiz', Health and Social Service Journal, 14 July

Halpern, S. (1985) 'What the Public Thinks of the NHS', Health and Social Service Journal, 6 June, pp. 702-704

Halpern, S. (1986) 'They Want More Money for the Health Service', Health Service Journal, 15 May, pp. 654-655

Halpern, S. (1987) 'Newton Wags the NHS Tail', Health Service Journal, Vol. 97, p. 301

Ham, C.J. (1980) 'Community Health Council Participation in the NHS Planning System', Social Policy and Administration, Vol. 14, no. 3, pp. 221-231

Ham, C.J. (1981) Policy Making in the National Health Service, London, Macmillan

Ham, C.J. (1982) Health Policy in Britain, London, Macmillan

Ham, C.J. (1985) Health Policy in Britain, London, Macmillan, 2nd edition

Ham, C.J. (1986) Managing Health Services: Health Authority Members in Search of a Role, Bristol, University of Bristol School for Advanced Urban Studies

Ham, C.J. & Hill, M.J. (1984) The Policy Process in the Modern Capitalist State, Brighton, Sussex, Wheatsheaf

Hambleton, R. (1986) Rethinking Policy Planning, Bristol, University of Bristol, School for Advanced Urban Studies

REFERENCES

Hampton, J.R. (1983) 'The End of Clinical Freedom',
British Medical Journal, Vol. 287, no. 6401,
pp. 1237-1238
Hardy, C. (1986) 'Management in the NHS: Using
Politics Effectively', Public Policy and
Administraton, Vol. 1, no. 1, pp. 1-17
Harrison, A. & Gretton, J. (eds) (1984) Health Care
UK 1984: An Economic, Social and Policy Audit,
London, Policy Journals
Harrison, S. (1981a) 'Health Service Work Roles and
the Pattern of Hospital Provision', Hospital
and Health Services Review, Vol. 77, no. 2, pp.
38-41
Harrison, S. (1981b) 'The Politics of Health
Manpower' in (eds) A.F. Long and G. Mercer,
Manpower Planning in the National Health
Service, Farnborough, Gower Press
Harrison, S. (1982) 'Consensus Decisionmaking in the
National Health Service: a Review', Journal of
Management Studies, Vol. 19, no. 4, pp. 377-
394
Harrison, S. (1984) 'Did Consensus Fail?, Senior
Nurse, Vol. 1, no. 2, 11 April, pp. 16-18
Harrison, S. (1986) 'Management Culture and
Management Budgets', Hospital and Health
Services Review, Vol. 82, no. 1
Harrison, S. (1988a) 'The Closed Shop and the
National Health Service: a Case Study in Public
Sector Labour Relations', Journal of Social
Policy, vol. 17, Pt. 1, pp. 61-81
Harrison, S. (1988b) 'The Workforce and the New
Managerialism' in R.J. Maxwell (ed.), Reshaping
the National Health Service, pp. 141-152,
Hermitage, Berks, Policy Journals
Harrison, S. & Hallas, J. (1979a) 'Political Skills
and the Science of Diplomacy', Health and
Social Service Journal, Vol. LXXXIX, no. 4668,
pp. 1486-1488
Harrison, S. & Hallas, J. (1979b) 'Politics and
Conjurers' Rabbits', Health and Social Service
Journal, Vol. LXXXIX, no. 4669, p. 1523
Harrison, S., Haywood, S. & Fussell, C. (1984a)
'Problems and Solutions: the Perceptions of
NHS Managers', Hospital and Health Services
Review, vol. 80, no. 4
Harrison, S., Pohlman, C.E. & Mercer, G. (1984b)
Concepts of Clinical Freedom Amongst English
Physicians, Paper presented at EAPHSS
Conference on Clinical Autonomy, King's Fund
Centre, 8 June

REFERENCES

Haywood, S.C. (1977) Decision Making in the New NHS:
  Consensus or Constipation?, London, King's Fund
  Project Paper no. 17
Haywood, S.C. (1979) 'Team Management in the NHS:
  What is it all About?', Health and Social
  Service Journal, Centre 8 Paper, 5 October
Haywood, S.C. (1983) District Health Authorities in
  Action, Birmingham, University of Birmingham,
  Health Services Management Centre, Research
  Report no. 19
Haywood, S.C. & Alaszewski, A. (1980) Crisis in the
  Health Service: the Politics of Management,
  London, Croom Helm
Haywood, S.C., Alaszewski, A., Elcock, H.J., James,
  T.L. & Law, E. (1979) The Curate's Egg... Good
  in Parts: Senior Officer Reflections on the
  NHS, Hull, University of Hull, Institute for
  Health Studies
Haywood, S.C. & Ranade, W. (1985) District Health
  Authorities in Action: Two Years On,
  Birmingham, University of Birmingham, Health
  Services Management Centre
Health Services Management Centre (1984)
  'Memorandum' in Social Services Committee First
  Report: Session 1983-84: Griffiths NHS
  Management Inquiry Report, pp. 179-182, London,
  House of Commons/HMSO
Heller, T. (1979) Restructuring the Health Service,
  London, Croom Helm
Henley, D., Holtham, C., Likierman, A. & Perrin,
  J.R. (1986) Public Sector Accounting and
  Financial Control, Wokingham, Van Nostrand
  Reinhold/CIPFA
Hennessy, P. (1987) 'Labour and Whitehall, Bridging
  the Ignorance Gap', New Statesman, 23 October,
  p. 14
Hildrew, P. (1987) 'Doctors Resist Undermining By
  Managers', Guardian, 30 June, p. 2
Hill, M.J. & Bramley, G. (1986) Analysing Social
  Policy, Oxford, Blackwell
Holmes, M. (1985) The First Thatcher Government,
  1979-1983: Contemporary Conservatism and
  Economic Change, Brighton, Wheatsheaf
Howell, R. (1982) 'National Health Service or
  Insatiable Master?', The Consultant, October,
  pp. 4-5
Hunter, D.J. (1979) 'Practice: Decisions and
  Resources in the National Health Service
  (Scotland)' in (ed.), K.M. Boyd, The Ethics of
  Resource Allocation in Health Care, Edinburgh,
  Edinburgh University Press

REFERENCES

Hunter, D.J. (1980) Coping with Uncertainty,
    Letchworth, Research Studies Press
Hunter, D.J. (1984) 'Managing Health Care', Social
    Policy and Administration, Vol. 18, no. 1, pp.
    41-67
Hunter, D.J. (1986) Managing the National Health
    Service in Scotland: Review and Assessment of
    Research Needs, Scottish Health Service Study
    no. 45, Edinburgh, Scottish Home and Health
    Department
Hyde, A. (1986) 'RGMs set to Discuss NHS National
    Plan', Health Service Journal, 3 July, p. 374
Institute of Health Services Management (1987)
    Memorandum to the Social Services Select
    Committee Inquiry into NHS Management, London,
    Mimeo
Jackson, P.M. (1985a) 'Policy Implementation and
    Monetarism: Two Primers' in P.M. Jackson
    (ed.) Implementing Government Policy
    Initiatives: The Thatcher Administration 1979-
    1983, London, Royal Institute of Public
    Administration
Jackson, P.M. (1985b) 'Perspectives on Practical
    Monetarism' in P.M. Jackson (ed.), Implementing
    Government Policy Initiatives: The Thatcher
    Administration 1979-1983, London, Royal
    Institute of Public Administration
Jaques, E. (1978) Health Services: Their Nature and
    Organisation and the Role of Patients, Doctors
    and the Health Professions, London, Heinemann
Jenkin, P. (1979) Letter of Baroness Robson of
    Kiddington, 2 August, Enclosed with DHSS Press
    Release no. 79/193
Jenkins, L., Bardsley, M., Coles, J., Wickings, I. &
    Leow, H. (1987) Use and Validity of NHS
    Performance Indicators - A National Survey,
    London, CASPE Research/King's Fund
Johnson, D. (1988) 'Doctor Gets Her Job Back',
    Guardian, 9 January, p. 3
Johnson, D.M. (1962) The British National Health
    Service: Friend or Frankenstein?, London,
    Johnson Publications
Johnson, P. (1986) 'Some Historical Dimensions of
    the Welfare State Crisis', Journal of Social
    Policy, Vol. 15, part 4, pp. 443-465
Johnson, T.J. (1972) Professions and Power, London,
    Macmillan
Joint Working Party (1967a) (Chairman: Mr G.P.E.
    Howard) The Shape of Hospital Management in
    1980?, London, King Edward's Hospital Fund for
    London

REFERENCES

Joint Working Party on the Organisation of Medical
    Work in Hospitals (1967b) (Chairman: Sir George
    Godber) First Report, ('The Cogwheel Report'),
    London, HMSO
Jones, T. & Prowle, M. (1984) Health Service
    Finance: an Introduction, London, 2nd edition,
    Certified Accountants Educational Trust
Jordan, A.G. & Richardson, J.J. (1987) British
    Politics and the Policy Process, London, Allen
    and Unwin
Kakabadse, A. (1982) Culture of the Social Services,
    Aldershot, Gower
Keegan, W. & Pennant-Rea, R. (1979) Who Runs the
    Economy? Control and Influence in British
    Economic Policy, London, Temple Smith
Keeling, D. (1972) Management in Government, London,
    Allen and Unwin
Keynes, J.M. (1936) The General Theory of
    Employment, Interest and Money, London,
    Macmillan
Kingdon, J.W. (1984) Agendas, Alternatives and
    Public Policies, Boston, Mass., Little, Brown
King's Fund Working Party (1977) (Chairman: Dr Bryan
    Thwaites) The Education and Training of Senior
    Managers in the National Health Service,
    London, King Edward's Hospital Fund for London
Klein, R.E. (1974) 'Policy Making in the National
    Health Service', Political Studies, Vol. 22,
    no. 1, pp. 1-14
Klein, R.E. (1978) 'Normansfield: Vacuum of
    Management in the NHS', British Medical
    Journal, Vol. ii, pp. 1802-1804
Klein, R.E. (1980) Ideology, Class and the National
    Health Service, Project Paper no. RC 4, London,
    King's Fund
Klein, R.E. (1983) The Politics of the National
    Health Service, London, Longman
Klein, R.E. (1984a) 'Who makes decisions in the
    NHS?', British Medical Journal, Vol. 288, no. 2
Klein, R.E. (1984b) 'The Politics of Ideology vs.
    the Reality of Politics: the Case of Britain's
    National Health Service in the 1980s', Millbank
    Memorial Fund Quarterly: Health and Society,
    Vol. 62, no. 1, pp. 82-109
Klein, R.E. (1985a) 'Management in Health Care: the
    Politics of Innovation', International Journal
    of Health Planning and Management', vol. 1, no.
    2, pp. 57-63
Klein, R.E. & Lewis, J. (1976) The Politics of
    Consumer Representation, London, Centre for
    Studies in Social Policy

REFERENCES

Kogan, M., Goodwin, B., Henkel, M., Korman, M.,
    Packwood, T., Bush, A., Hoyes, V., Ash, L. &
    Tester, J. (1978) The Working of the National
    Health Service, Royal Commission on the
    National Health Service, Research Paper no. 1,
    London, HMSO
Kotter, J.P. (1982) The General Managers, New York,
    Free Press
Krieger, J. (1986) Reagan, Thatcher and the Politics
    of Decline, Cambridge, Polity Press
Lamb, S.M. & David, T.J. (1985) 'Playing with Fire:
    an Experiment in Clinical Budgeting', British
    Medical Journal, Vol. 290, pp. 650-651
Larson, L.L., Bussom, R.S., Vicars, W. & Jauch
    (1986) 'Proactive versus Reactive Manager: Is
    the Dichotomy Realistic?', Journal of
    Management Studies, Vol. 23, no. 4, pp. 385-
    400
Lee, K. & Mills, A. (1982) Policy-Making and
    Planning in the Health Sector, London, Croom
    Helm
Levitt, R. (1979) The Reorganised National Health
    Service, 2nd edition, London, Croom Helm
Levitt, R. & Wall, A. (1984) The Reorganised
    National Health Service, London, Croom Helm
Lewis, J. (1986) What Price Community Medicine? The
    Philosophy, Practice and Politics of Public
    Health Since 1919, Brighton, Wheatsheaf
Lindblom, C.E. (1959) 'The Science of Muddling
    Through', Public Administration Review, Vol.
    19, no. 3, pp. 79-88
Lindblom, C.E. (1979) 'Still Muddling, Not Yet
    Through', Public Administration Review, Vol.
    39, no. 6, pp. 517-526
Lindsey, A. (1962) Socialised Medicine in England
    and Wales: The National Health Service 1948-
    1961, Chapel Hill, NC, University of North
    Carolina Press
Linstead, D. (1984) 'The Realities of Human
    Resourcing: a Case Study which Questions the
    Utility of Rational Manpower Planning Models in
    Health Care', Health Services Manpower Review,
    Vol. 10, no. 3, pp. 9-11
Lipsky, M. (1980) Street-Level Bureaucracy, New
    York, Russell Sage Foundation
Long, A.F., Harrison, S. & Mercer, G. (1985)
    'Comparative Perspectives on Performance' in
    A.F. Long and S. Harrison (eds), Health
    Services Performance: Effectiveness and
    Efficiency, London, Croom Helm

REFERENCES

Long, A.F., Mercer, G., Brooks, F., Harrison, S.,
Rathwell, T. & Barnard, K. (1987) Health
Manpower: Planning, Production and Management,
London, Croom Helm
Ludbrooke, A. & Mooney, G.H. (1984) 'Clinical
Freedom, Efficiency and The Griffiths Report',
British Medical Journal, Vol. 288, pp. 420-421
MacGregor, S. (1985) 'Making Sense of Social
Security' in P.M. Jackson (ed.), Implementing
Government Policy Initiatives: The Thatcher
Administration 1979-1983, London, Royal
Institute of Public Administration
Mangham, I.L. (1979) The Politics of Organisational
Change, London, Associated Business Press
Majone, G. (1986) 'Mutual Adjustment by Debate and
Persuasion' in F.X. Kaufmann, G. Majone and V.
Ostrom (eds), Guidance Control and Evaluation
in the Public Sector: the Bielefeld
Interdisciplinary Project, Berlin, Walter de
Gruyter
Maynard, A. & Bosanquet, N. (1986) Public
Expenditure on the NHS: Recent Trends and
Future Problems, London, Institute of Health
Services Management (in association with
British Medical Association and Royal College
of Nursing)
McKay, D. & Cox, A. (1978) 'Confusion and Reality in
Public Policy: the Case of the British Urban
Programme', Political Studies, Vol. XXVI, no.
4, pp. 491-506
Medical Services Review Committee (1962) (Chairman:
Sir Arthur Porritt) A Review of Medical
Services in Great Britain, London, Social
Assay
Miliband, R. (1977) Marxism and Politics, Oxford,
Oxford University Press
Millar, B. (1987a) 'Options on Community Care',
Health Service Journal, Vol. 97, no. 5065, p.
984
Millar, B. (1987b) 'Doctors Want Debate on
Inadequate Acute Funding', Health Service
Journal, Vol. 97, p. 1426
Mills, I. (1987) 'Regional Realism: Reaping
Rewards', Health Service Journal, 23 April, pp.
470-471
Ministry of Health (1962) National Health Service: A
Hospital Plan for England and Wales, Cmnd 1604,
London, HMSO
Ministry of Health and Department of Health for
Scotland (1944) A National Health Service, Cmnd
6502, London, HMSO

REFERENCES

Ministry of Health and Scottish Home and Health
    Department (1966) Report of the Committee on
    Senior Nursing Staff Structure, (Chairman: Mr
    Brian Salmon) London, HMSO
Mintzberg, H. (1973) The Nature of Managerial Work,
    New York, Harper and Row
Mintzberg, H. (1979) The Structuring of
    Organisations, Englewood Clifs, NJ, Prentice
    Hall
Moore, W. (1987a) 'RHA Refuses to Take Part in
    Public Inquiry on Funds', Health Service
    Journal, 23 April, p. 464
Moore, W. (1987b) 'Doctors in Scotland Complain to
    Department', Health Service Journal, 30 July,
    p. 864
Moore, W. (1987c) 'Paradox of Cutting Waiting
    Lists', Health Service Journal, 7 May, p. 523
Nairne, P. (1983) 'Managing the DHSS Elephant:
    Reflections on a Giant Department', Political
    Quarterly, Vol. 54, no. 3, pp. 243-256
Nairne, P. (1985) 'Managing the National Health
    Service', British Medical Journal, Vol. 291,
    pp. 121-124
National Audit Office (1986) Report by the
    Comptroller and Auditor General: Value for
    Money Developments in the National Health
    Service, London, HMSO
National Board for Prices & Incomes (1967) The Pay
    and Conditions of Manual Workers in Local
    Authorities, the National Health Service, Gas
    and Water Supply, Report no. 29, London, HMSO
National Health Service Management Inquiry (1983)
    Report ('The Griffiths Report'), London,
    Department of Health & Social Security
National Health Service Training Authority (1986)
    Developing the Role of Doctors in the
    Management of the National Health Service: A
    Discussion Document, Bristol
Naylor, W.M. (1971) Organisation and Management of a
    Unified Health Service: Organisation of Area
    Health Services, London, Institute of Health
    Service Administrators
Oakley, R. & Wood, N. (1988) 'GPs Could Opt Out of
    NHS in Shake-Up Plan: Private Health Care Key
    to Government Thinking', The Times, 23
    February, p. 1
O'Connor, J. (1973) The Financial Crisis of the
    State, New York, St Martin's Press
Offe, C. (1984) Contradictions of the Welfare State,
    (edited and translated by J. Keane), London,
    Hutchinson

REFERENCES

O'Higgins, M. (1984) 'Computerising the Social
    Security System: An Operational Strategy in
    Lieu of a Policy Strategy?', Public
    Administration, Vol. 62, no. 2, pp. 201-210
Pater, J.E. (1981) The Making of the National Health
    Service, London, King's Fund
Peach, L. (1987) 'NHS Managers', Letter to the
    Editor, IPM Digest, no. 265, p. 4
Petchey, R. (1986) 'The Griffiths Reorganisation of
    the National Health Service: Fowlerism by
    Stealth?', Critical Social Policy, Vol. 6, no.
    2, pp. 87-101
Peters, T.J. & Waterman, R.H. (1982) In Search of
    Excellence, New York, Harper and Row
Pettigrew, A.M. (1973) The Politics of
    Organisational Decisionmaking, London,
    Tavistock
Pettigrew, A.M. (1985) The Awakening Giant:
    Continuty and Change in Imperial Chemical
    Industries, Oxford, Blackwell
Pfeffer, J. (1978) Organistional Design, Arlington
    Heights, Ill., AHM Publishing Corporation
Pfeffer, J. (1981) Power in Organisations,
    Marshfield, Mass., Pitman
Pfeffer, J. & Salancik, G.R. (1978) The External
    Control of Organisations: A Resource Dependence
    Perspective, New York, Harper and Row
Pollitt, C.J. (1984a) 'Professionals and Public
    Policy', Public Administration Bulletin, no.
    44, pp. 29-41
Pollitt, C.J. (1984b) Manipulating the Machine:
    Changing the Pattern of Ministerial Departments
    1960-83, London, Allen and Unwin
Pollitt, C.J. (1985a) 'Measuring Performance: A New
    System for the National Health Service', Policy
    and Politics, Vol. 13, no. 1, pp. 1-15
Pollitt, C.J. (1985b) 'Can Practice be Made
    Perfect?', Health and Social Service Journal, 6
    June, pp. 706-707
Pollitt, C.J. (1986) 'Beyond the Managerial Model:
    the Case for Broadening Performance Assessment
    in Government and the Public Services',
    Financial Accountability and Management, Vol.
    2, no. 3, pp. 155-170
Pollitt, C.J., Harrison, S., Hunter, D.J. & Marnoch,
    G. (1988) 'The Reluctant Managers: Clinicians
    and Budgets in the NHS', Financial
    Accountability and Management, Vol. 4, no. 3

REFERENCES

Polsby, N.W. (1980) Community Power and Political
    Theory: A Further Look at Problems of Evidence
    and Inference, 2nd edition, New Haven CT, Yale
    University Press
Popper, K.R. (1972) Objective Knowledge: An
    Evolutionary Approach, Oxford, Oxford
    University Press
Pugh, D.S. & Hickson, D.J. (1976) Organisational
    Structure in its Context, Farnborough, Saxon
    House
Rathwell, T.A. (1987) Strategic Planning in the
    Health Sector, London, Croom Helm
Rathwell, T. & Barnard, K. (1985) 'Health Services
    Performance in Britain' in A.F. Long and S.
    Harrison (eds), Health Services Performance:
    Effectiveness and Efficiency, London, Croom
    Helm
Richards, T. (1986) 'HMOs: America Today, Britain
    Tomorrow?', British Medical Journal, Vol. 292,
    pp. 460-463
Roberts, F. (1952) The Cost of Health, London,
    Turnstile Press
Robinson, A. (1985) 'The Financial Work of the
    Select Committees' in G. Drewry (ed.), The New
    Select Committees: A Study of the 1979 Reforms,
    pp. 307-318, Oxford, Clarendon Press
Robinson, A. & Webb A. (1987) Parliamentary
    Responses to the Government's Efficiency and
    Effectiveness Initiatives, Paper presented to
    the JUC Public Administration Committee, York,
    7 September
Robinson, R. (1986) 'Restructuring the Welfare
    State: An Analysis of Public Expenditure
    1979/80 to 1984/85', Journal of Social Policy,
    Vol. 15, Part 1, pp. 1-21.
Rodrigues, J.M. (1987) 'DRGs: the European Scene - a
    General Analysis', Journal of Management in
    Medicine, Vol. 2, no. 2, pp. 139-150
Rowbottom, R.W., Balle, J., Cang, S., Dixon, M.,
    Jaques, E., Packwood, T. & Tolliday, H. (1973)
    Hospital Organisation, London, Heinemann
Royal Commission on the National Health Service
    (1979) (Chairman: Sir Alec Merrison) Report,
    Cmnd 7615, London, HMSO
Rush, M. (1985) 'The Social Services Committee' in
    G. Drewry (ed.), The New Select Committees: A
    Study of the 1979 Reforms, pp. 307-318, Oxford,
    Clarendon Press
Sarlvik, B. & Crewe, I. (1983) Decade of
    Dealignment, Cambridge, Cambridge University
    Press

REFERENCES

Saunders, P. (1986) Social Theory and the Urban Question, London, Hutchinson, 2nd edition

Schulz, R.I. & Harrison, S. (1983) Teams and Top Managers in the NHS: a Survey and a Strategy, London, King's Fund Project Paper no. 41

Schulz, R.I. & Harrison, S. (1986) 'Physician Autonomy in the Federal Republic of Germany, Great Britain, and the United States', International Journal of Health Planning and Management, Vol. 1, no. 5, pp. 335-355

Schulz, R.I. & Scheckler, W.E. (1988) Physician Concerns and Experiences with the Incorporation of Health Maintenance Organisations into Private Practice, mimeo, Dept of Preventive Medicine, University of Wisconsin - Madison

Scottish Health Services Council (1966) (Chairman: Mr W.M. Farquharson-Lang) Administrative Practice of Hospital Boards in Scotland, Edinburgh, HMSO

Scottish Home and Health Department (1985) General Management in the Scottish Health Service: Implementation - the First Steps, Circular 1985 (GEN) 4

Scottish Home and Health Department (1986) General Management at Unit Level and the Development of Senior Management Structures, Circular 1986 (GEN) 20

Scrivens, E. (1987) The Management of Clinicians in the Hospitals of the English National Health Service, Paper presented at EAPHSS Conference, Utrecht, 17 June

SDP/Liberal Alliance (1987) United for Britain - the Time Has Come: The SDP/Liberal Alliance Programme for Government, London

Seldon, A. (ed.) (1980) The Litmus Papers: A National Health Dis-service, London, Centre for Policy Studies

Shaw, C.D. (1986) 'Time to Close Up the Quality Gap', Health and Social Service Journal, 23 January, pp. 110-111

Sherman, J. (1985) 'The Power Struggle for UGM Posts', Health and Social Service Journal, 7 February, p. 152

Shortell, S.M., Becker, S. & Neuhauser, D. (1976), 'The Effects of Management Practices on Hospital Efficiency and Quality of Care' in Organisation Research in Hospitals, Chicago, Blue Cross Association

Simon, H.A. (1957a) Administrative Behaviour, New York, Macmillan, 2nd edition

Simon, H.A. (1957b) Models of Man, New York, Wiley

REFERENCES

Simon, H.A. (1959) 'Theories of Decision Making in Economics and Behavioural Science', American Economic Review, XLIV, June

Smith, A. (1987) 'Clinical Freedom', British Medical Journal, Vol. 295, p. 1583

Social Services Committee (1980) Third Report, Session 1979-80: The Government's White Papers on Public Expenditure: the Social Services (in two volumes), London, House of Commons/HSMO

Social Services Committee (1981) Third Report, Session 1980-81: Public Expenditure on the Social Services (in two volumes), London, House of Commons/HMSO

Social Services Committee (1982) Third Report, Session 1981-82: 1982 White Paper: Public Expenditure on the Social Services (in two volumes), HC 306, London, House of Commons/HMSO

Social Services Committee (1984) First Report, Session 1983-84: Griffiths NHS Management Inquiry Report, HC209, London, House of Commons/HMSO

Social Services Committee (1986) Fourth Report, Session 1985-86: Public Expenditure on the Social Services (in two volumes), London, House of Commons/HMSO

Solesbury, W. (1976) 'The Environment Agenda: An Illustration of how situations may become political issues and issues may demand responses from government: or how they may not', Public Administration, Vol. 54, pp. 379-397

Steering Group on Health Services Information (1982) (Chairman [sic]: Mrs E Korner) First Report to the Secretary of State, London, HMSO

Stewart, J.S.S. (1984) 'Budgeting for Griffiths', British Medical Journal, Vol. 288, pp. 731-732

Stewart, J. (1979) The Reality of Management, London, Pan Books

Stewart, R., Gabbay, J., Dopson, S., Smith, P. & Williams, D.T.E. (1987) Managing with Doctors: Working Together?, Issue Study no. 5, Oxford, Templeton College

Stewart, R., Smith, P., Blake, J. & Wingate, P. (1980), The District Administrator in the National Health Service, London, King's Fund

Stocking, B. (1985) Initiative and Inertia: Case Studies in the NHS, London, Nuffield Provincial Hospitals Trust

Stowe, K. (1986) 'Managing a Great Department of State', Journal of the Royal Society of Arts, No. 5363, Vol. CXXXIV, pp. 731-741

REFERENCES

Syrett M. (1986) 'NHS Management: Here to Stay?',
    Manpower Policy and Practice, Winter, pp. 10-11
Taylor, D. (1984) Understanding the NHS in the
    1980s, London, Office of Home Economics
Taylor-Gooby, P. (1985a) 'Attitudes to Welfare',
    Journal of Social Policy, Vol. 14, Pt. 1, pp.
    73-81
Taylor-Gooby, P. (1985b) Public Opinion, Ideology
    and State Welfare, London, Routledge and Kegan
    Paul
Taylor-Gooby, P. & Dale, J. (1981) Social Theory and
    Social Welfare, London, Edward Arnold
Thain, C. (1985) 'The Education of the Treasury: the
    Medium-Term Financial Strategy 1980-84', Public
    Administration, Vol. 63, no. 3, pp. 261-285
Thompson, D.J.C. (1986) Coalition and Decision-
    Making Within Health Districts, Research Report
    no. 23, Birmingham, University of Birmingham,
    Health Services Management Centre
Timmins, N. (1985) 'And May the Best Man Be Vetoed',
    The Times, 21 January
Timmins, N. (1988) 'Health Finance: the Options',
    The Independent, 8 February, p. 3
Timmins, N. & Brown, C. (1987) 'Government to Launch
    Major Review of the NHS', The Independent, 17
    December, p. 1
Tolliday, H. (1978) 'Clinical Autonomy' in E.
    Jacques (ed.), Health Services: their nature
    and organisation and the role of patients,
    doctors, and the health professions, London,
    Heinemann
Y Travis, A. (1986) 'And It's Goodbye to the Fall
    Guys', Health Service Journal, 18 September, p.
    1219
Tynedale, G. (1987) 'Newton Backs Down on GP
    Practice Allowance', Health Service Journal, 1
    January 1987, p. 6
Ward, H. (1987) 'Structural Power - A Contradiction
    in Terms?', Political Studies, Vol. XXXV, pp.
    593-610
Warden, J. (1987) 'Long Run of Short Reports',
    British Medical Journal, Vol. 294, p. 1299
Wassenberg, A. (1977) 'The Powerlessness of
    Organisation Theory' in S. Clegg and D.
    Dunkerley (eds), Critical Issues in
    Organisations, London, Routledge and Kegan
    Paul
Watkin, B. (1975) Documents on Health and Social
    Services: 1834 to the Present Day, London,
    Methuen

REFERENCES

Watkin, B. (1978) The National Health Service: The
First Phase - 1948-1974 and After, London,
Allen and Unwin
Webb, N.L. & Wybrow, R.J. (1981) The Gallup Report,
London, Sphere Books
Welsh Office (1984a) NHS Management Inquiry Report:
Implementation in Wales, Circular WHC(84)15
Welsh Office (1984b) NHS Management Inquiry:
Implementation in Wales, Circlar WHC(84)22
Wilks, S. (1985) 'Conservative Industrial Policy
1979-83' in P.M. Jackson (ed.), Implementing
Government Policy Initiatives: The Thatcher
Administration 1979-1983, London, Royal
Institute of Public Administration
Willcocks, A.J. (1967) The Creation of the National
Health Service, London, Routledge and Kegan
Paul
Williams, A.H. (n.d.) Medical Ethics: Health Service
Efficiency and Clinical Freedom, Nuffield/York
Portfolio no. 2, London, Nuffield Provincial
Hospitals Trust
Wintour, P. & Wheen, F. (1982) 'The Knives are Out',
New Statesman, 15 October, pp. 8-10
Wiseman, C. (1979) 'Strategic Planning in the
Scottish Health Service - A Mixed - Scanning
Approach', Long Range Planning, Vol. 12, Pt. 2,
pp. 103-113
Working Party on Medical Administrators (1972)
(Chairman: Dr R.B. Hunter) Report, London,
HMSO
✗Yates, J. (1983) 'When Will the Players Get
Involved?', Health and Social Service Journal,
15 September, pp. 1111-1112
Young, K. (1977) 'Values in the Policy Process',
Policy and Politics, Vol. 5, pp. 1-22
Young, K. & Mills, L. (1983) Managing the Post-
Industrial City, London, Heinemann

INDEX